Keto Meal Prep

*Lose Weight, Save Time and Money
While On a Ketogenic Diet (A Guide
for Beginners and Intermediates)*

Alexandros Costa

Table of Contents

Introduction

Welcome to *Keto Meal Prep*!

The following chapters will "dissect" everything that you need to know to get started with using meal prep to make the ketogenic diet easier. While the ketogenic diet is a great plan to go on to help you lose more weight and make you feel better overall, it can sometimes be hard to implement it in daily life. You may worry about sticking with this diet when you are busy, have to stay late at work, or when you are dealing with those pesky cravings. Meal prepping can be the answer you are looking for.

This guidebook is going to spend some time talking about meal prepping and helping you get started. We will talk about some of the basics of meal prepping, why people choose to meal prep, how it can save you time and money, and the basic steps that you must follow to be successful with meal prepping. We will also include some tasty recipes, including breakfast, lunch, dinner, and those quick options that you need on-the-go.

When you are on the ketogenic diet, and you want to ensure that you are giving yourself the best chance of success no matter what, make sure to check out this guidebook and learn how meal prepping can help you out!

There are plenty of books on this subject on the market, thanks again for choosing this one! Every effort was made to ensure it is full of as much useful information as possible, please enjoy!

Chapter 1:
Introduction

Why Meal Prepping?

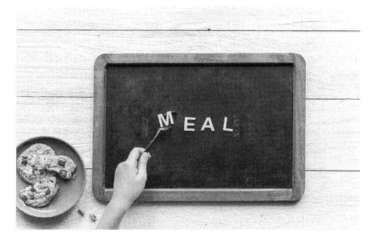

There are so many reasons why you are going to fall in love with meal prepping. So many people are already falling in love with meal prepping because it allows them to always have healthy and cost-effective meals around even when they are busy. And if you are on the ketogenic diet, you will find that the meal prepping process is more important than ever. Some of the reasons why you may choose to get started with meal prepping include:

- *Meal prepping can help you stay on your diet plan*

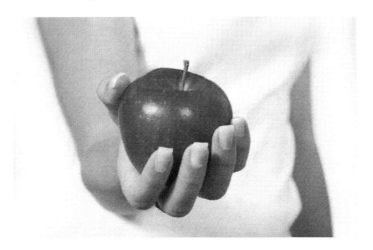

Meal prepping is a great way to ensure that you stay on your diet plan, especially the ketogenic diet. Many times, we get busy during the week. When we get to those nights that we don't have a lot of time, it is hard to stick with a diet plan. When it comes to a diet plan that eliminates some of those fast and easy foods we enjoy, like the ketogenic diet does, then it becomes even more difficult to stick without best goals.

Many people fail with their diet because they don't have a plan. They get tired of coming up with diet approved meals at the last minute when they are tired. They find that they have nothing prepared. So, they have to go out to eat, and they splurge.

Meal prepping can help solve some of these problems. You can pick a day of the week, perhaps the weekend, where you are less stressed-out and have some time. Then, you go and prepare all of the meals that you need during the week. When it comes to the ketogenic diet, it's a good idea to plan for breakfast, lunch, dinner, and dessert.

When you meal prep, you are able to sit down and plan out each of your meals. You can decide if they have enough nutrients in them if you are getting the macronutrients you need, and you are better prepared to know whether you are sticking with the diet or not. And since you are doing this ahead of time, you don't have to worry about being too tired or stressed out after work when you do this.

Once the meals are done, you can just grab them and go for the rest of the week. You won't have to worry about whether they fit the ketogenic diet or not because you figured this out ahead of time. You reduce some of the stress, take out some of the guesswork, and make it much easier for you to stick with the ketogenic diet compared to someone who doesn't meal prep.

- *Meal prepping can save you money*

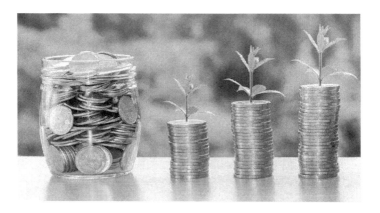

A big reason that a lot of people decide to start with meal prepping is that they want to save money. Eating out can get expensive. Feeding a cheap meal to a family of four at a fast food restaurant can easily cost you $30 or more each time you do it. If you get busy and need to do this for two or three times a week, it can cost you hundreds of dollars each month.

Some families also run into the issue of wasting money on food they don't use. If you have the best intentions of making a meal with some healthy ingredients but then you run out of time to make it, and the ingredients go bad, you can waste a lot of money as well.

Meal prepping can really help out with this. If you have some healthy meals that are already prepared at home, then you are less likely to run out to eat on those busy nights. You can just pop the meal in the oven or the slow cooker, and you are ready to go. It doesn't take you any more time, but since you can make a big casserole with leftovers for $5 to $10, you have already saved a lot of money.

Many people who meal prep decides to freeze their meals as well. This allows them to make those healthy dinners with lots of vegetables inside without worrying about the produce going bad. When you prep these ahead of time, they fit nicely into the freezer and are ready to go whenever you need them, even if you don't pull them out for a few weeks. This can also help save you a lot of money.

- *Meal prepping can save you time*

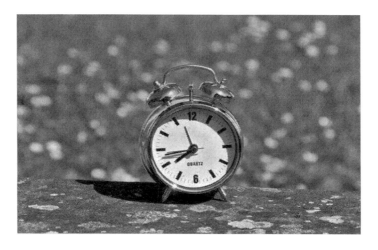

Many of us don't have the time necessary to make a healthy and nutritious meal every night for our families. We have all the best intentions, but there are some nights when we have to run to sports and practices and so much more. By the time we get home, it may be almost bedtime which can make it really hard to get a meal, and everyone will be tired and hungry.

Even on those nights when you just went straight home from work, you can be too tired to think of cooking a big meal for your family. You just want to find something that is quick and nutritious and will fill everyone up.

Meal prepping is a great option because it can ensure that you have those healthy and satisfying meals ready whenever you want. Whether you are busy or too tired or something else comes up, the meals are already pre-planned for you and ready to go.

And since you batched cooked (meaning you made several of the same meals at the same time), you saved a lot of time. Making one big thing of the same meal rather than just making a small version can save you money and provides you two meals in the time it usually takes you to do it once.

Many people choose to work on meal prepping over the weekend. This makes it easier for them to have some free time to do the work, and then they can relax during the week. Either way, it can end up saving you a lot of time while still ensuring that you eat healthily, save money, and feed your family.

What is Meal Prepping?

Meal prepping is one of the best things that you can do for your sanity. It is the act of preparing some, or even all, of your meals ahead of when you need them. Think about how easy it is to go to the store and pick out a TV dinner. You can just grab it out of the freezer whenever you want, throw it in the microwave, and enjoy on those busy nights.

Meal prepping is just like that, other than it costs a lot less money and is much healthier than those TV dinners. You simply pick out the meals that you want to cook, prepare them, and then throw them in the freezer. Then, whenever you need them, you pull them out and cook up what is needed before enjoying.

Not only can this save you time, but it also helps you to eat healthier foods and keeps you in proper portions. For families that are constantly busy with work, school and other obligations, it can be a lifesaver to ensure that a healthy and delicious supper gets on the table without having to resort to going to the local fast food restaurant.

All of us have those busy days when we just don't have the time to make a meal. We want to save money and eat healthier, but when there is no time to cook until 9 p.m. or later, it just seems impossible. Most of us resort to unhealthy choices including snacks and meals when we end up in this situation.

With meal prepping, you won't have to deal with this decision. You can have the meals ready to go ahead of time so that when one of those busy nights shows up, you have a ready-made meal to enjoy. It's convenient, it saves you money, and it can still bring the family together.

There are many different ways to go about meal prepping. Some people choose to prepare all of their food for the week over the weekend. This can help when you are on a diet plan and want to know ahead of time that your meals will fit the dietary recommendations of the diet plan you chose. Then throughout the week, you just grab the meal that you need and go.

Others choose to just meal prep a few meals at a time. They know that they occasionally run into those busy nights or they have those days when work is hard, and they just want a day off from cooking. They may prepare some meals ahead of time and then pull them out of the freezer when needed.

The good news is that you can't do meal prepping the wrong way. As long as you make sure that the meals are healthy and cost-effective, and you choose those options on your busy nights instead of something unhealthy, then you are succeeding!

This guidebook is going to focus on options that you can do for meal prepping that are simple to make, delicious, fast, and have cheap ingredients that you can find at your local grocery store. Meal prepping doesn't have to be complicated. In fact, it's supposed to be simple. Follow this guidebook to see just how much easier meal prepping can make your life!

Chapter 2:
Alexandros' Meal Prepping Map to Success – Meal Prepping Essentials

Now that you know a little bit more about meal prepping and some of the benefits of using it, it is time to understand how to get started. This chapter is going to spend some time mapping out exactly what you need so that you can really get going with meal prepping even as a beginner. We will talk about the equipment that you need for meal prepping, how to store the food, how to pick a day to start, and how to pack the items. Let's get started by taking a look at each of these categories.

Equipment Needed for Meal Prepping

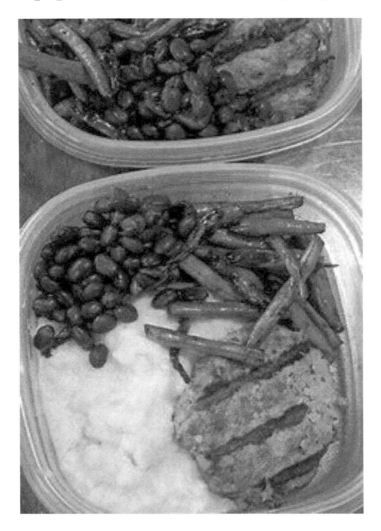

Having the right equipment when you get started with meal prepping is going to make all the difference. Luckily, meal prepping is not going to require a ton of items to help you out. Some of the best equipment that you should get for meal prepping in your home includes:

- **Grocery list:** Eating healthy is going to start when you hit the grocery store. You want to make sure that you go in there armed with a list of all the things that you need. It doesn't have to be complicated. Just make sure that your list includes all the ingredients that you must have for your recipes. It can help you save time, ensures you don't waste time at the store, and helps keep you on a healthy diet.

- **Food scale:** When it comes to meal prepping, portion size can be really important. A food scale is going to help you find out the right size for all the foods that you eat. Make sure to find one that is high-quality and that fits into your own budget.

- **Measuring cups:** One of the easiest ways for you to eat healthier is to use some measuring cups. Eyeballing how much of something you add to a dish may seem simple, but it leaves you with no idea of how much of something is there. With measuring cups, you can maintain proper portion control throughout.

- **Sharp knives:** There will be plenty of times that you will need to slice up things to get going with meal prepping. Having a sharp knife is the best because it can speed up the process and will keep you safer.

- **Cutting board:** You can't properly cut into or slice something without a good cutting board. You may find that it is best to have a few cutting boards; one for meats and another for your produce. This ensures that you don't end up with cross-contamination of the foods.

- **Flavored oils and seasonings:** You will be surprised at how much a simple spice or herb can change a whole dish. Having some variety of spices in your pantry can make a big difference.

Flavored oils, as long as there are no added sugars in them, can help as well.

- **Slow cooker:** The slow cooker is going to make a big difference in meal prepping. Nothing is easier than throwing some ingredients in the slow cooker in the morning and coming home to some amazing meals. Explore the different brands to see what is available for your needs.

- **Containers:** You will need something to put all your meals into when you are done and when you take them with you to work. Consider what containers you are most likely to use for meal prepping and then purchase some high-quality ones to make this easier.

What and When to Prepare

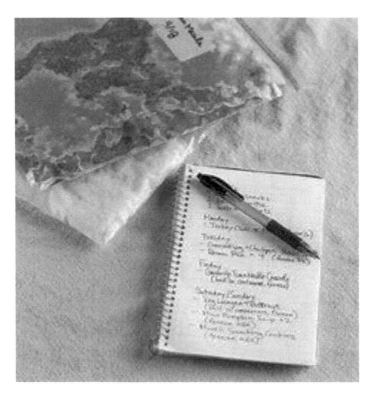

The first thing to consider is when you should prepare your meals. The answer is going to vary for each person. You want to go on a day of the week when you aren't at work and when you won't be stressed out with the work that needs to be done. You will probably need at least a few hours to get things prepped for the week, so pick out a day that will allow you to do this.

Many people like to go on Sunday afternoon to do this. They can have the whole afternoon to get the work done and go to bed that night knowing that all their meals for the week are ready. But if you work weekends, you may need to pick out another day that works better. Just make sure that you go with the day that works the best for you.

When it comes to what you should prepare with meal planning, prepare as much meal ahead of time as possible. The less work you have to do when it's time to eat the meal later in the week, the better. This means that you can chop up the vegetables, make the sauces, cook up what you can, and get the meat cooked up (unless you are grilling, then you can save this for later).

Most of these meals will end up in the freezer later on so that you can heat them up when you are ready. Even those that go in the fridge to cook later can get quite a bit done ahead of time. Think ahead when planning meals on what you could do to reduce the workload later that week. If something can be done ahead of time, then it is in your best interest to get it done.

Some tips on what you can work on ahead of time when it comes to meal prepping include:

- Cook up the meat

- Slice the vegetables and cook those up

- Prepare the sauces

- Assemble the casseroles

- Add in the spices

- Throw ingredients in a bag for freezer meals.

How to Store

There are different ways that you are able to store the meals you make. If you are only making a few days of food at a time, you may choose to put them in the fridge. Ensure that you put the stuff that you are going to eat first at the front and then slowly start bringing things up as you use them.

Another popular option, especially if you are making a week or more of meals at a time, is to use the freezer. This helps to keep the food fresh for as long as you need it, and if any plans change, nothing will go bad. There are a ton of recipes that do well with freezing so look for some of those and add them into your meal prep schedule.

How to Pack

After the meals and the ingredients are done, you will want to make sure that you pack up everything properly. This will ensure that you have all the right nutrients in place and that you won't get hungry when you head out the door for the day. You can also do this as part of your meal prepping when you do all the work on Sunday (or whichever day works the best for you).

You will want to make sure that you have a good protein, plenty of fresh produce, and a snack to help you get through the day. With the ketogenic diet, the macronutrients are so important, so try to plan this out ahead of time. You can write down exactly what needs to go with you each day or what needs to be served on each dinner. This takes out some of the guesswork but ensures that you are going to be set for the whole day.

Things to Remember When Packing

- **Don't forget the snacks:** Before you head out the door, make sure that you pack up at least a few snacks. It is likely that you will get hungry at some point during the day. And if you only bring something to eat during lunch time, you are going to be scrambling for something, later on, to keep you full. Unfortunately, it's likely that the snack you do choose is going to be something unhealthy. Instead of falling into that trap, consider bringing along some healthy snacks to keep you happy.

- **Include some protein:** Every meal needs to have a good source of protein. This helps to keep the muscles strong, and they often come with some good sources of fats that the ketogenic diet desires.

- **Keep the majority as the produce**: A good source of protein is great to include when packing your meals but make sure that there is plenty of great produce. This helps to fill you up and will ensure that you don't take on too many carbs during the day while on the ketogenic diet.

- **Plan out the packing ahead of time:** Trying to remember what goes with each meal when you are tired or in a hurry can be a challenge. A better option would be to plan this out ahead of time. For example, you can start on Monday and write out everything that you need for breakfast, everything that needs to go with you for lunch, and what you will need to pull out for dinner. This may sound silly, but it can really help you out on many nights.

Chapter 3:
How to Save Time and
Meal Prep Fast

One of the best benefits of meal prepping is that it can save you a lot of time and can give you a ton of meals for the whole week for a good price. But you have to be efficient and pay attention to what you are doing to ensure that meal prepping is fast and will actually save you time when it comes to making your meals. Some of the tips that you can use to save time and get meal prepping done fast for the whole week include:

- **Pick a day that works for you**

Before you get started with meal prepping, you need to pick out a day of the week that works the best for you. Don't try to do this sometime after work. You will simply be too tired to even do a good job. It is better to pick out a day when you can give your whole focus and attention to the endeavor because that will make it go much faster and can make the experience more enjoyable.

If you are busy, it is fine to pick out a day every two weeks that works for you. The great thing about meal prepping is that you can make it work for your schedule. Many people find that grocery shopping on Saturday and then doing the actual cooking on Sunday works the best for them. But if you get days off in the middle of the week or seem to work better on Monday, then pick this day.

- **Do meals that have similar ingredients**

If possible, consider finding recipes that have similar ingredients. You can then prepare all these ingredients at the same time rather than doing them one at a time. If you have a few recipes that have chicken, you can cook the chicken all at once rather than just the amount that you need for one recipe. If you have recipes that need certain vegetables, you can slice them all up at the same time instead of going back and forth.

Meals that have similar ingredients can make it easier to prepare. It can also save you money. You will be able to purchase the ingredients in bulk which always saves you money. You can choose to go on a theme to make the meals similar, or you can choose that one week will be chicken, and the next week hamburger, and so on.

- **Consider freezer meals**

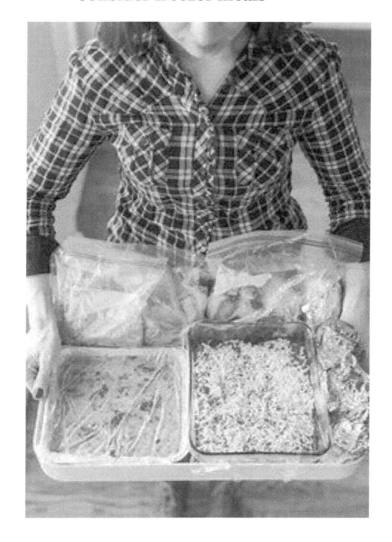

Freezer meals can be a great way to meal prep. Often, you will be able to throw the ingredients in a casserole dish or into a freezer bag, and they are ready to go. Make these meals slow cooker or dump dinner ideas, and you are really going to be able to meal prep in no time.

Some freezer meals are going to take a little bit of time for you to put together. You will have to make up the casserole before putting it in the freezer to use later. There are also many great options that just ask for a few ingredients to be thrown into a bag. This will only take you a few minutes to prepare, and then you can add them to the air fryer or even the slow cooker when it is time to eat that meal later on.

- **Work on meals together, not one at a time**

A common mistake that you can make is to cook each meal on its own. If you are doing this, then you are not saving any time at all. It is best if you can cook meals at the same time. Most meals don't need your full attention while you are doing them. For example, zoodles take some time to cook so you can work on something else at the same time.

If you have several recipes that need zoodles or the same meat, cook all that you need at once. It will take about the same amount of time and can make completing the meals faster than ever. When the noodles are done, for example, you can then add them to all the meals that need them before storing them.

- **Don't wait for things**

If the noodles are cooking, the vegetable is cooking, or the meat is cooking, don't stand around and wait for them to get done. Look through the recipe and find out what you can be working on in the meantime. Consider what vegetables need to be sliced, what sauces you can combine, and anything else that needs to go in the dish. That way, when the meat, zoodles, or other ingredients are done, you can add them to the casserole dish or other container and then store them to eat later on.

To get meal prepping done as quickly as possible, you need to keep moving the whole time. Have a plan for what things to start first, what things can be done at the same time, and what will take the longest so that you can get the work done quickly without wasting any time.

- **Batch-make meals**

Don't waste your time making just one of each meal. A good meal prep recipe will be easy to double or triple the recipe. In the same amount of time, you could make the same meal three or four times and then freeze what you are not using right away. Have ten recipes that you really like to use for each meal and then triple them. In a fraction of the time, you will have a months' worth of meals, and it didn't take you near as long.

The main reason that a lot of people are fond of meal prep is that they are able to get delicious and nutritious meals cooked up in a fraction of the time. Follow some of these simple tips, and you will be able to enjoy some tasty meals in no time as well.

Chapter 4:
How to Save Money with Meal Prepping

When it comes to meal planning, you want to make sure that you are saving as much money as possible. All of us want to ensure that we are not spending more money than we have to on our meals, and with the ketogenic diet, you want to be even more careful about this. With the help of some of these great tips, you are going to be able to save a ton of money when you meal prep using the ketogenic diet.

- **Pick out meals that keep well**

You want to pick out meals that are either going to keep well in the fridge or that you can freeze. This can ensure that you are not throwing out a lot of good food and will save you money over time. There are a lot of great meals that you can cook up and then freeze for later. Consider working with a few of those each week so that you are always prepared and don't have to worry about throwing out good food.

- **Consider using your slow cooker**

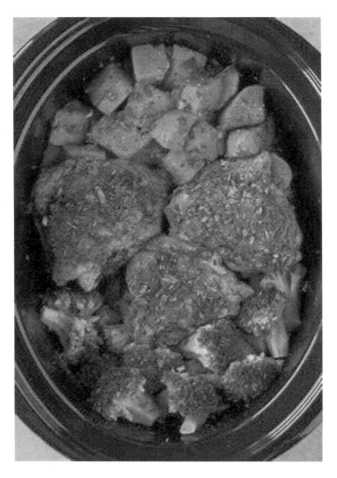

A slow cooker is a great tool when it comes to meal prepping. It can cook up many of your favorite meals and adds a new twist to them.

There are many reasons why you will fall in love with your slow cooker when it comes to meal prepping including:

- **Takes things from frozen to cooked:** Meal prepping with a slow cooker is easy. You can take frozen items and add them in, and everything will be cooked by the end of the day. You don't have to prepare a ton of items ahead of time.

- **Put the food in at the beginning of the day:** You can throw a few items into the slow cooker in the morning and then when you get home, the items will all be cooked through. Saves you time and who doesn't like a healthy and delicious meal when they get home from work.

- **Makes big meals:** There are many different sizes when it comes to slow cookers. You can easily get a large one and fill it up, doubling a recipe if needed. When you are done for the night, you can use the leftovers the next day or freeze them to add to next weeks' meal prepping.

- **Label everything**

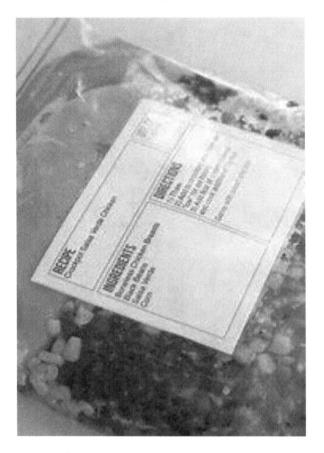

Meal prepping isn't going to do you much good if you can't remember what is in each dish. Once they get put into the fridge or even the freezer, it can be hard to remember what is inside each one. Something could get pushed to the bottom of the freezer and forgotten, costing you money. Or you might get so frustrated with trying to remember what is in each container that you give up and order something to eat.

When it comes to labeling, make sure that you write out what is inside each container as well as the date that it was made. This can make it easier to know how old each item is and can ensure that you always eat things at the right time before it goes bad.

- **Stick with reusable containers**

Don't waste your time on containers and cooking pans that should be thrown away after one or two uses. Sure, these are often cheaper in the beginning than the traditional pans, but if you have to replace them a few times a month, that is going to add up.

Consider investing in some good containers and casserole dishes, and anything else you will need for meal prepping. This can cost you a little bit extra when you first start. But since you just need to clean them before reusing them, the costs will quickly go down, and you will end up saving money in the long run.

- **Double all the recipes**

When you are making a recipe, consider doubling it. This is going to save you time and money in the long run. You can spend the same amount of time cooking that one meal, but you get the benefit of putting two of it in the freezer. Buying a big can of marinara sauce and a big size of low carb noodles to split between two pans is going to cost less than making that meal two separate times.

When you are writing out your meal plan, consider whether you can make the same meal twice during the week or plan out two weeks ahead of time and double up the recipe. If not, consider if you can use the leftovers of one recipe in the new one, or if there are two similar recipes where you can purchase the same ingredients in bulk. This will help you reduce costs when you are at the store and ensures that you don't waste time when preparing the meals.

- **Visit the farmer's market at night**

Going to the farmer's market is a great way to save money when you are meal prepping. But if you wait and go at the end of the day, when all the vendors are ready to head home, you can save a lot more money. Most of these vendors are going to want to get rid of the produce, so they don't have to bring it home and it doesn't go bad. This means that you can get a great deal on the food you need. Sure, the best looking produce may not be left, but even the bruised food is delicious and has all the same nutrition.

After you get back from the farmer's market, you can prepare that produce right away. Freezing, steaming, and roasting are good options to help you prepare your new fruits and veggies to have on hand when you need them. Take care of them right away. It is not saving you a lot of money if you end up throwing away all the produce you bought.

- **One night a week is a leftover night.**

When you create your meal plan, you should consider setting aside one night a week where you try to use up everything that is leftover all at once. You can bring out everything and let your family pick out some of their favorites. You can search through the fridge and find items that are almost done and don't have a lot left or items that may not last long in the fridge. This can make sure that you are not throwing away good food and wasting it, and can give you a night off from actually cooking.

• Cut out the meat a few nights a week

The parts of your meals that are probably the most expensive are the cuts of meats. While these are great on the ketogenic diet and can really help to fill you up, the more meat that you have on your meal plan, the more expensive it will be. A good way to help you to save some money when you are creating a meal plan is to cut out meat. There are a lot of vegetarian options that you can go with that are healthy and will fit with the ketogenic diet. It can also save you a ton. Consider making one or two nights a week vegetarian and see what a difference it can make in your overall grocery bill.

• Go with dried beans

Dried beans are really cheap. They do take you a little bit longer to prep compared to working with the canned variety, but you are going to notice a big difference when it comes to how much you spend. You can add these dried beans to a slow cooker, and there are a ton of recipes that are based on chickpeas and black beans. Add in that the dried varieties of beans are way lower in sodium, and you have a great option that is really cheap.

- **Plan meals centered around eggs**

As someone on the ketogenic diet, rejoice in knowing that you can make a lot of different meals with the help of eggs. A carton of a dozen eggs usually costs under $1.50 in most stores, and it can help you make a lot of meals for very little. Add in some vegetables or make some traditional meals with this as the protein, and you are set to go for very little.

There are a ton of options for breakfast, lunch, dinner, and even snacks when it comes to using eggs. You can consider breakfast tacos with scrambled eggs, avocado toast with a soft boiled egg, a green salad with a poached egg and so much more. Revel in the fact that not only will these eggs save you money; they are also a really easy way to fill you up and add in the protein that your body needs to stay healthy.

Saving money is one of the main goals of working with meal prepping. With some good planning and knowing which meals to cook, you are sure to save as much money as possible while also enjoying some easy and satisfying meals.

Chapter 5:
How to Lose Up To 2 Extra Pounds Per Week with Meal Prepping

Many people who go on a diet plan are looking to do so not only to improve their health but to help them lose weight. They are tired of holding onto the extra pounds, and they want a simple and stress-free way to get rid of the weight as quickly as possible.

The cool thing about meal prepping is that it can help you lose weight faster than ever. With less stress, pre-portioned out servings, and the choice of snacks and other things that you need to eat during the day, you are sure to see some great results in no time. When you add on the ketogenic diet, you are sure to see some amazing results faster than ever.

If you are ready to start losing weight and want to see how meal prepping can make it easier, and even help you to lose an extra two pounds per week compared to just dieting all on its own, take a look below. These are some of the great ways that meal prepping is going to help you become the best version of you possible with some great weight loss!

- **Reduces the stress**

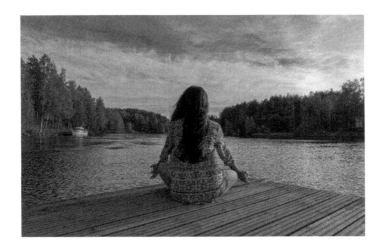

Meal prepping is going to reduce the amount of stress that you feel. Think about all those times when it is getting late, and you start to stress out about what meal you will make for dinner that night. Thanks to the stress hormones, when you do finally figure out what to make, it is more likely that you will eat too much. Add in that the stress hormones will make you store all those extra calories you just ate in your fat cells, and it can become almost impossible for you to lose the weight you want.

When you go with meal prepping, this stress can go away. You already know what you are going to eat each day and you don't have to stress about it each day. Think of how nice it would be to come home each night and just throw something in the oven without thinking about it. You can let it cook while you get changed and start relaxing. This already reduces the amount of stress you have and can help to keep those harmful hormones out of the way when you eat.

- **Cuts down on your reliance on willpower**

On many diets, you need to rely on your own willpower. They want you to be able to resist overeating or eating only certain foods in limited amounts. Some even expect that you will be able to ignore nearly constant hunger pains. This can be a challenge even for the most dedicated person, and they can all be reasons that someone is going to fail in their diet plans.

You can take all of these things out of the equation when you go with meal prepping. You will know ahead of time that you have good meals and snacks to enjoy all day. As long as you pick options that are healthy, well-balanced, and satisfying, you will feel like you are getting little treats throughout the day, rather than having to use your willpower to help you get through.

- **Keeps you away from the drive-thru**

This is a big reason why a lot of people will go with meal prepping. There are so many bad things about going to the drive-thru. First, it is expensive. Feeding a family of four can cost you $30 or more each time that you go. You can easily make a handful of meals with meal prepping for this amount.

In addition, the foods at these restaurants are often loaded with bad fats, carbs, and lots of calories. One meal there can really throw you over your calorie count and still leave you feeling hungry within a few hours. Most of these restaurants don't include healthy options, especially ketogenic-approved options, so you are throwing your weight loss goals out the window. Do this a few times a week, and it can be really hard to lose weight.

Meal prepping can help you break this cycle. You will have these meals ready when you come home at the end of the day, taking away the stress and ensuring that everyone has something to eat even when you are running short on time or energy. This is much healthier and can really help you cut down on that weight. If you were a frequent visitor to fast food restaurants before starting with meal prep, you are sure to see a huge increase in the amount of weight you will lose simply by cutting out the fast food.

- **Better help with portion control**

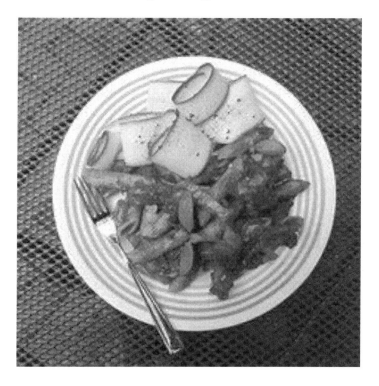

If you are struggling with your weight loss goals, the issue may be portion control. If you are worried about how much you eat at each meal, you can take the time to divide your meal preps into individual servings. This ensures that you don't eat too much when it is time to enjoy your efforts and can help you keep your calories in check.

You may need to experiment with this a little bit. Some people will only need small servings to feel full and satisfied while others may do fine with bigger portions if they are more active. Learn how to listen to your body on this one. Only eat as much as you are hungry for, not necessarily as much as in the container. This will help you know what the right portion is for you.

- **Prepping your snacks can avoid mindless munching.**

One big culprit that stops your weight loss goals is mindless munching. Healthy snacking can be a really good thing. It can help control your hunger and can reduce the amount of cravings that you have for sugar. However, if you don't take proper care of your snacking, it is one of the easiest ways to take in too many carbs and too many calories which will ruin your weight loss goals.

This is where meal prepping can help. You can make some of your own snacks ahead of time. When you do this, you can portion out your snacks to make sure that they are healthier and that you won't take on too many carbs or calories all at once. And when you know exactly what kinds and amounts of snacks you can have, you will be less likely to just munch on anything random in the house. You can enjoy the sliced vegetables all that you want, but be careful about how much fruits, seeds, and nuts you have between meals when you put together your snacks.

- **Meal prepping can give you more time to relax and sleep**

It is hard to lose weight if you don't get enough sleep. Sleep is a quality of weight loss that a lot of people forget about. They might work hard to eat the right types and amounts of food and try to stay active. But then they end up only getting a few hours of sleep a night and wonder why they struggle with losing weight.

When you don't get enough sleep at night, your weight loss goals will struggle. Poor sleep habits have been shown to increase food cravings and can cause you to eat more than you should on days that you don't get enough sleep.

When you meal prep, you won't have to struggle with getting meals on the table each night. You can even go to sleep a little earlier. Plus, you will always have healthy meals on hand so you won't have to worry about giving into those bad cravings.

- **Meal prep and exercise results in more fat loss**

When you combine regular exercise with a good routine of meal prep, you are really going to kick out those fat cells faster than ever before. You will use the exercise in order to get your body revved up and ready to go. And then, you will fill your body with healthy meals that can keep that fat loss going. Both exercising and good meal prepping are going to require some discipline on your part. But when you combine them together, the results are going to be amazing, and you will lose a ton of weight.

- **Prep with your friends to make it a friendly competition**

To help you lose more weight, you can grab a family member or another friend who wants to lose weight as well. You both can decide to cook your meals together or have a competition to see who is able to come up with the best meals out of the two. You can even trade the dishes that you prep to add in some more variety and to keep meal prepping more interesting.

In addition, the real advantage of working on meal prepping with a friend is to support and inspire each other. You both can ensure that you are staying on the ketogenic diet and can push each other to lose even more weight with meal prepping.

While meal prepping can make it much easier to eat healthier meals and to save money, it can also make it so much easier to lose the weight that you want. And with the right meal prepping techniques, you can lose an extra two pounds per week compared to not using any type of meal prepping.

Chapter 6:
How to Kick-Start Your Day – Easy Ketogenic Breakfast Meal Ideas

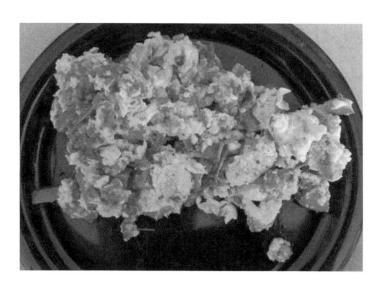

Spicy Scramble

Servings: 2

Serving Size: half the egg mixture

What's inside:

- Pepper
- Salt
- Whipping cream, heavy (2 Tbsp.)

- Eggs (6)
- Spicy sausage (6 oz.)
- Ghee (2 Tbsp.)
- Chopped scallions (.5 cup)
- Shredded cheese (.5 cup)

How to make:

1. Start this by bringing out a skillet and melting the ghee on it. Add the sausage and brown it for the next six minutes to cook through.

2. While that cooks, you can throw the eggs inside and make it frothy. Then, add in the pepper, salt, and cream and whisk well.

3. Make sure that the skillet keeps the fat inside and push the sausage over. Add the egg mixture to the other side and cook it for another three minutes to cook almost through.

4. When these eggs are close to done, mix in some of the shredded cheese. Then,

combine the sausage and eggs and top with the rest of the scallions and cheese.

5. Spoon onto two plates and serve warm.

Nutrients:

- Fat: 70g
- Protein: 46g
- Carbs 7g
- Net Carbs 6g

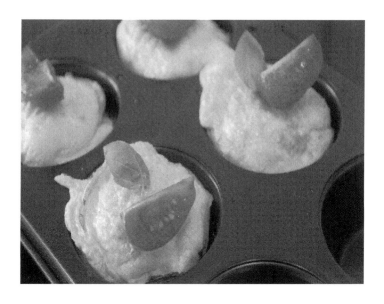

Egg Cups with Bacon

Servings: 6

Serving Size: 1 egg cup

What's inside:

- Bacon
- Butter (1 Tbsp.)
- Bacon slices (6)
- Eggs
- Cream cheese (2 oz.)
- Eggs (4)

- Jalapeno peppers (2)
- Cheese (.25 cup)
- Pepper
- Salt

How to make:

1. Turn on the oven and give it time to heat up to 375 degrees. While this oven warms up, heat up a skillet on the stove.

2. When the skillet is hot, add in some butter to grease it up before adding the bacon slices. Partially cook them for the next four minutes. Move to a plate that is lined with a paper towel.

3. Coat some muffin tin cups with butter and then place the bacon in these cups to line the sides.

4. Now you can work on the eggs. Cut the jalapeno and seed and mince it. Cut the rest into rings and set aside.

5. Now, you can use a hand mixer to beat the eggs. Add in the jalapeno and cream cheese and season this.

6. Pour this into the muffin tin with the bacon. Make sure to leave a little room on top for this to rise. Top with some cheese and jalapeno and then place in the oven.

7. After 20 minutes, take the cups out and let them cool down before serving.

Nutrients:

- Fat: 13g
- Protein: 9g
- Carbs: 1g
- Net Carbs: 0g

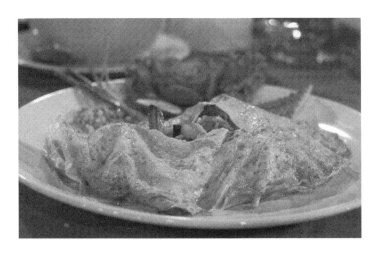

Bacon and Spinach Egg Wrap

Servings: 2

Serving Size: 1 wrap

What's inside:

- Pepper
- Salt
- Whipping cream, heavy (2 Tbsp.)
- Eggs (2)
- Bacon slices (6)
- Sliced avocado (.5)
- Spinach (1 cup)
- Butter (1 Tbsp.)

How to make:

1. Bring out your skillet and let the bacon cook for eight minutes to make it crispy. Then, add this prepared bacon to a plate with some paper towels.

2. Take out a bowl and make sure to whisk the eggs well with the pepper, salt, and cream.

3. Add half of this new mixture into the pan with the bacon grease. Let this cook for a little bit until it sets.

4. When it sets, you can flip this around and cook for another minute. Move this to a plate with a paper towel.

5. Repeat these steps to get the other half of your eggs cooked. You can add in a little butter if the pan starts to get dry.

6. Place this egg mixture on two warmed plates. Top each of these with some avocado slices, bacon, and spinach.

7. Season with pepper and salt and roll up these wraps before serving.

Nutrients:

- Fat: 29g
- Protein: 17g
- Carbs: 5g
- Net Carbs: 2g

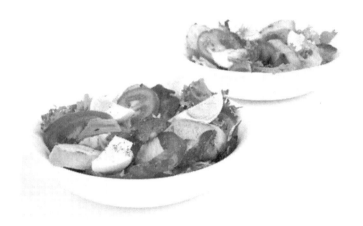

BLT Morning Salad

Servings: 2

Serving Size: half the salad mixture

What's inside:

- Chopped bacon slices (6)
- Halved grape tomatoes (5)
- Sliced avocado (1)
- Pepper
- Salt
- Olive oil (2 Tbsp.)
- Mixed greens (5 oz.)
- Eggs (2)

How to make:

1. Take out a pan and fill it up with some water. Let this boil before adding in the eggs to soft boil. You can then turn the heat down and let these cook for a bit.

2. When the eggs are cooling, you can toss the mixed greens together with the pepper, salt, and olive oil. Divide up the greens into two bowls.

3. Top this with the bacon, grape tomatoes, and slices of avocado.

4. Once the eggs get done, you can peel them, cut them in half, and then place two halves on top of each salad before serving.

Nutrients:

- Fat: 39g
- Protein: 18g
- Carbs: 19g
- Net Carbs: 4g

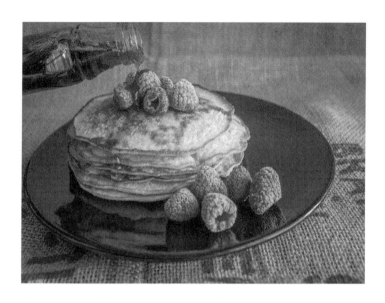

Cream Cheese Pancakes

Servings: 2

Serving size: 3r pancakes

What's inside:

- Baking powder (1.5 tsp.)
- Liquid stevia (1 tsp.)
- Cream cheese (4 oz.)
- Butter (4 Tbsp.)
- Coconut flour (4 Tbsp.)

How to make:

1. Bring out the blender or a food processor. You can add in the coconut flour, baking powder, stevia, cream cheese, eggs and blend well.

2. Take out your skillet and melt some butter on it. Pour a bit of the batter onto the skillet so that you end up with three at a time.

3. You will see that the pancakes start looking puffy when it's time to flip them. Cook for another minute and then take off the skillet.

4. Repeat the steps again with the rest of the batter including the butter and then serve these warm.

Nutrients:

- Fat: 55g
- Protein: 36g
- Carbs: 13g
- Net Carbs: 8g

Breakfast Quesadilla

Serves: 2

Serving Size: 1/2 quesadilla

What's inside:

- Low carb, tortillas (2)
- Olive oil (1 Tbsp.)
- Pepper
- Salt
- Eggs (2)
- Slices of bacon (2)
- Sliced avocado (.5)
- Cheese, shredded (1 cup)

How to make:

1. This one will need a skillet heated up. Then, you can add on the bacon and cook to make crispy.

2. Move the cooked bacon to a plate with paper towels on it and then cool down. When this is cool, you can chop up the bacon on a cutting board.

3. Turn the heat on the skillet down a bit and then crack your eggs into that bacon grease. Season how you like with some pepper and salt.

4. Cook these for a bit so the egg whites can set. When you feel that they are done, you can move to a plate.

5. Pour some olive oil into the skillet and add in the tortilla to this pan. Add in half a cup of cheese and add the avocado slices on top of this.

6. Top with the fried eggs, the chopped bacon, and the rest of the cheese. Cover with the second tortilla.

7. When the cheese melts and the tortilla is golden, flip it over. Cook for a bit longer.

8. Slice up the quesadilla and then serve.

Nutrients:

- Fat: 41g
- Protein: 27g

- Carbs: 27g
- Net Carbs: 9g

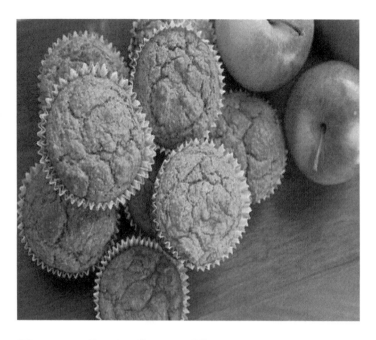

Heavenly Soft Muffins

Serves 6

Serving Size: 1 muffin

What's inside:

- Mexican blend cheese (1 handful)
- Cream cheese (2 oz.)
- Heavy cream (2 Tbsp.)
- Beaten eggs (2)
- Baking powder (.75 Tbsp.)

- Almond flour (1 cup)
- Melted butter (4 Tbsp.)

How to make:

1. Turn on the oven and allow it time to heat up to 400 degrees. While that heats up, you can take some butter and coat the muffin tin.

2. Now, you will want to mix the baking powder and almond flour in a bowl.

3. In a second bowl, mix the eggs, cream cheese, heavy cream, butter, and shredded cheese together.

4. Pour your flour mixture in with this and then use your hand mixer to beat it well.

5. Pour this batter into your muffin cups. Place these into the warm oven to bake.

6. After 12 minutes, the muffins are done. Take them out of the oven and let them cool before serving.

Nutrients:

- Fat: 23g
- Protein: 8g
- Carb: 6g
- Net Carbs: 4g

Chapter 7:
Meal Prepping Ideas for
Lunch and Dinner

Poultry Meals

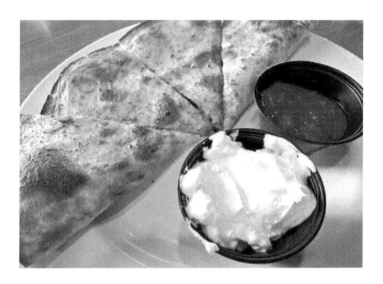

Chicken Quesadilla

Servings: 2

Serving size: ½ quesadilla

What's inside:

- Shredded chicken (2 oz.)

- Cheese blend, shredded (.5 cup)
- Low carb tortillas (2)
- Olive oil (1 Tbsp.)
- Sour cream (2 Tbsp.)
- Tajin seasoning salt (1 tsp.)

How to make:

1. Bring out a skillet and heat up the olive oil. Add a tortilla to this skillet and top with some of the cheese, the chicken, the Tajin seasoning, and then the rest of the cheese.

2. Top all of these ingredients with the second tortilla. Let these cook. Pay attention to how the cheese is melting and whether or not the tortilla is browning.

3. After a few minutes, you can flip this quesadilla over. Give it another minute to finish.

4. Move this all to a cutting board and let it cool down. Cut into four pieces and then put two pieces onto each plate. Top with some sour cream before serving.

Nutrients:

- Fat: 28 g
- Protein: 26g
- Carbs: 24g
- Net Carbs: 7g

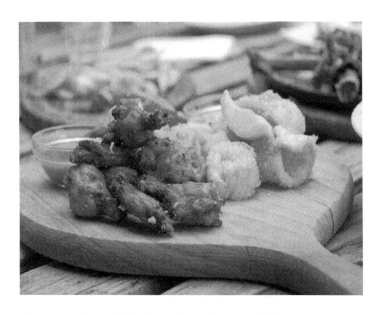

Saturday Night Chicken Wings

Servings: 4

Serving Size: .25 pounds chicken wings

What's inside:

- Chicken wings: 1 lb.)
- Pepper
- Salt
- Parmesan cheese (.25 cup)
- Italian seasoning, dried (1 Tbsp.)
- Minced garlic cloves (2)

- Butter (8 Tbsp.)

How to make:

1. Bring out your slow cooker and get it warmed up. You can then line up a baking sheet with the help of aluminum foil.

2. Put the parmesan cheese, Italian seasoning, garlic, and butter into the slow cooker and season with the pepper and salt.

3. Let the butter have some time to melt in the warmed-up slow cooker and then mix the ingredients together.

4. When this happens, add in the chicken wings and stir them around to be coated with butter.

5. Put the lid on the slow cooker and let this cook for three hours on a high setting.

6. Turn on the broiler of your oven and then move the prepared wings to your baking sheet. Sprinkle the rest of the cheese and add this to the broiler.

7. After five minutes, you can serve the wings.

Nutrients:

- Fat: 33g
- Protein: 20g
- Carbs: 2g
- Net Carbs: 2g

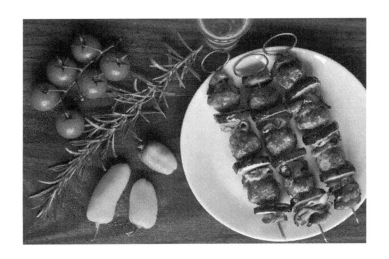

Chicken Skewers

Servings: 4

Serving size: 1 skewer

What's inside:

- Pepper
- Salt
- Peanut butter (2 Tbsp.)
- Toasted sesame oil (3 tsp.)
- Sriracha sauce (.5 tsp.)
- Soy sauce (3 Tbsp.)
- Cubed chicken breasts (1 lb.)

How to make:

1. Bring out your zip-lock bag, and combine your chicken with some of the soy sauce, half a teaspoon of sriracha sauce, and two teaspoons of the sesame oil.

2. Seal up the bag and make sure that the chicken gets to marinate for at least an hour. You can do this overnight as well.

3. Take out a big skillet and turn it up. Use the ghee to oil up the skillet.

4. While the skillet heats up, thread the chicken onto the skewers and then place onto the skillet for a bit.

5. After 15 minutes, the skewers are done. Remember to flip them around in the middle.

6. While those cook, you can mix the peanut dipping sauce. Stir the rest of the soy sauce, Sriracha sauce, sesame oil, and peanut butter together.

7. Serve this peanut sauce with the chicken skewers and enjoy.

Nutrients:

- Fat: 15g
- Protein: 31g
- Carbs: 3g
- Net carbs: 2.5g

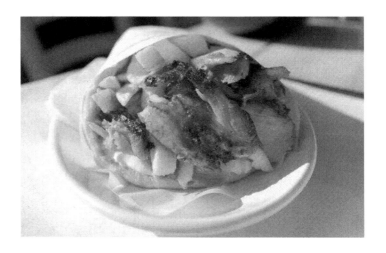

Easy Greek Chicken

Servings: 4

Serving Size: 1 chicken thigh

What's inside:

- Pepper
- Salt
- Chicken thighs (4)
- Butter (2 Tbsp.)
- Kalamata olives, pitted (.5 cup)
- Lemon (1)
- Chicken broth (.5 cup)
- Ghee (2 Tbsp.)

How to make:

1. Turn on the oven and let it heat up to 375 degrees. Use some paper towels to pat the chicken dry and then season with the pepper and the salt.

2. Take out a skillet and melt the ghee. Once the ghee is hot and melted, add the chicken thighs inside. Leave these for a bit, so the skin has time to get browned and crispy.

3. Flip the chicken at this time and cook a bit on the other side. While those finish, pour the chicken broth and add in the lemon juice, lemon slices, and olives.

4. Add this to the oven and let it bake for some time. After 30 minutes, you can take the chicken out.

5. Add butter to the broth mixture. Divide the chicken and the olives between four plates and serve.

Nutrients:

- Fat: 23g
- Protein: 14g
- Carbs: 2g
- Net Carbs: 1g

Cheesy Bacon and Chicken Casserole

Servings: 2

Serving Size: 1 chicken breast

What's inside:

- Cheddar cheese, shredded (.5 cup)
- Broccoli florets (2 cups)
- Cream cheese (6 oz.)
- Bacon slices (4)
- Pepper
- Salt
- Chicken breasts (2)
- Ghee (2 Tbsp.)

How to make:

1. Take the time to let the oven heat up to 375 degrees. Pick a big baking dish and coat it with the ghee.

2. Now, bring out the chicken breast and pat it dry with some paper towels. Then, you can season with pepper and salt.

3. Put the chicken breasts into the baking dish along with bacon slices. Place this in the oven.

4. After 25 minutes, you can take the chicken out of the oven and then use a fork to shred it up. You can also move the bacon out of the pan and crumble it up.

5. In a bowl, mix the broccoli, chicken, cream cheese, and half the bacon crumbles. Move the chicken mixture over to the baking dish and top with the cheese, and the rest of the bacon crumbles.

6. Add this baking dish into the oven and let it bake for a bit longer until it becomes browned and bubbling. About 35 minutes later, you can take the baking dish out of the oven and let it cool down before serving.

Nutrients:

- Fat: 66g
- Protein: 75g

- Carbs: 10g
- Net Carbs: 8g

Creamy Chicken in the Slow Cooker

Servings: 4

Serving Size: ½ chicken breast

What's inside:

- Spinach (2 cups)
- Pepper
- Salt
- Parmesan cheese (.25 cup)
- Sun-dried tomatoes (.25 cup)
- Alfredo Sauce (1 cup)
- Chicken breasts (2)
- Ghee (1 Tbsp.)

How to make:

1. For this recipe, bring out a skillet and melt the ghee on it. After the ghee is warm, add in the chicken and let it cook to get both of its sides browned and warm.

2. Take out your slow cooker and move the chicken over into it. Set the slow cooker to the low setting.

3. You will need to use a small bowl to combine the Parmesan cheese, sun-dried tomatoes, and Alfredo sauce. Season this with the salt and the pepper.

4. Pour this sauce over the chicken. Add the lid to the slow cooker and let this cook for the next four hours. You can check to see if the chicken is done after this time.

5. Add in the spinach and cook this just a bit longer to let the spinach wilt before serving.

Nutrients:

- Fat: 33g
- Protein: 35g
- Carbs: 4.5g
- Net Carbs: 3.5g

Fish and Seafood Meals

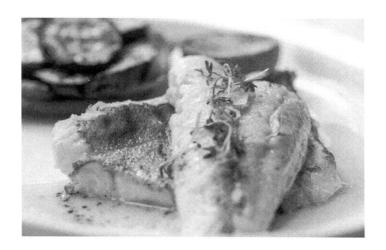

Baked Lemon Fish

Servings: 2

Serving Size: 1 fillet

What's inside:

- Rinsed and chopped capers (2 Tbsp.)
- Zested juiced lemon (1)
- Minced garlic cloves (2)
- Pepper
- Salt
- Tilapia fillets (2)

- Butter (4 Tbsp.)

How to make:

1. Turn on the oven and allow it to heat up to 400 degrees. Use your butter to help grease up a baking dish.

2. Pat the tilapia dry with some paper towels and then season with the pepper and salt. Place this into the baking dish.

3. Now, you need to bring out a skillet and melt the butter in it. Add in the garlic and cook this for about five minutes, allowing it to brown a bit but not burnt.

4. Take the garlic butter out of the heat and mix with the lemon zest and a few tablespoons of lemon juice.

5. Pour this over the fish and then sprinkle the capers all around the pan. Place the dish into the oven.

6. After 15 minutes, the fish should be cooked through, and you can take it out of the oven. Serve warm.

Nutrients:

- Fat: 26g
- Protein: 16g
- Carbs: 5g
- Net Carbs: 3g

Taco Bowl

Servings: 2

Serving Size: 1 bowl

What's inside:

- Salt
- Mashed avocado (1)
- Spicy Red Pepper Miso Mayo (1 Tbsp.)
- Coleslaw cabbage mix, sliced (2 cups)
- Tajin seasoning salt (4 tsp.)
- Olive oil (1 Tbsp.)
- Tilapia fillets (2)
- Pepper

How to make:

1. Turn on the oven and let it heat up to 425 degrees. Take out a baking sheet and line it with some aluminum foil.

2. Now, you can take some tilapia and rub olive oil all over it. Then coat with some of the Tajin seasoning salt and add to the prepared pan and place in the oven.

3. After 15 minutes, the fish should be cooked. You can take it out of the oven to cool down.

4. While that cools down, gently mix together the mayo sauce and coleslaw before adding in the rest of the Tajin sauce and the avocado. Season with pepper and salt.

5. Divide this between two bowls. Using two forks, shred up the prepared fish into pieces and place on your bowls.

6. Top with some of the mayo sauce and then serve.

Nutrients:

- Fat: 24g
- Protein: 16g
- Carbs: 12g
- Net Carbs: 5g

A Taste of the Sea Scallops

Servings: 4

Serving Size: 2 scallops

What's inside:

- Salt
- Parmesan cheese (.25 cup)
- Butter (1 Tbsp.)
- Whipping cream, heavy (1 cup)
- Bacon slices (4)
- See scallops (8)
- Ghee (1 Tbsp.)
- Pepper

How to make:

1. Bring out your skillet and cook the bacon on it for a bit to make the meat nice and crispy. Once cooked, place it on a plate that is lined with paper towels.

2. Lower the heat a bit. Then, add in the parmesan cheese, butter, and cream to the bacon-greased pan and season with the pepper and the salt to your liking.

3. Reduce the heat a bit, stirring the whole time until you get a nice thick sauce. This can take up to ten minutes.

4. In a second skillet, add the ghee and heat it up. Season your scallops a bit and then add them to the skillet. These only need to cook for 60 seconds on each side.

5. Move these cooked scallops to a plate lined with paper towels.

6. Divide up the cream sauce on two plates and then crumble the cooked bacon on top. Top everything with four scallops and then serve this meal right away.

Nutrients:

- Fat: 35g
- Protein: 12g
- Carbs: 6g
- Net Carbs: 5g

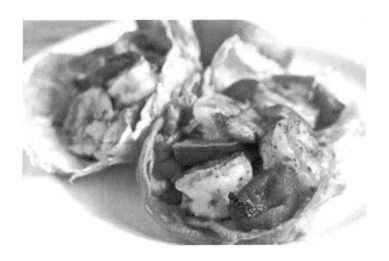

Shrimp Lettuce Cups

Serves: 2

Serving Size: 2 lettuce cups

What's inside:

- Shrimp (.5 lbs.)
- Ghee (1 Tbsp.)
- Spicy Red Pepper Miso Mayo (1 Tbsp.)
- Lettuce leaves, butter (4)
- Pepper
- Salt
- Sliced avocado (.5)
- Grape tomatoes (.5 cup)

How to make:

1. Bring out your skillet and heat up the ghee on it. When this is hot, you can add the shrimp to the skillet and cook it through.

2. Season with some pepper and salt and cook until the shrimps are pink and well-cooked.

3. Season the avocado and the tomatoes. Then, divide up your lettuce cups between two plates.

4. Fill up these cups with the avocado, tomatoes, and shrimp. Add the mayo sauce to the top and then serve.

Nutrients:

- Fat: 11g
- Protein: 33g
- Carbs: 7g
- Net Carbs: 4g

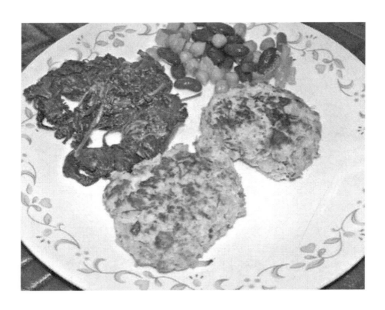

Salmon Cakes

Servings: 2

Serving Size: 2 patties

What's inside:

- Dijon mustard (.5 Tbsp.)
- Ghee (1 Tbsp.)
- Pepper
- Salt
- Mayonnaise (3 Tbsp.)
- Beaten egg (1)

- Pork rinds (2 Tbsp.)
- Alaska salmon (6 oz.)

How to make:

1. For this recipe, you can take out a bowl and combine a bit of the mayo with the egg, pork rinds, and salmon. Season all of these ingredients with the pepper and the salt.

2. Form four patties out of these cakes. Keep patting these patties to make sure they stick together well.

3. Now, bring out your skillet and let the ghee have some time to melt inside. When the ghee starts to sizzle, add your salmon patties inside so they can cook.

4. Cook these for three minutes on each side until browned. When they are done, move the patties over to a plate that is lined with paper towels.

5. While those cool down, mix the rest of the mayo with the mustard. Serve your salmon cakes with this mayo and mustard dipping sauce.

Nutrients:

- Fat: 31g
- Protein: 24g
- Carbs: 1g
- Net carbs: 1g

Meat Recipes

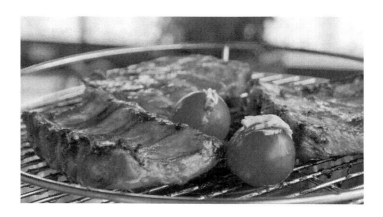

BBQ Ribs

Serves: 4

Serving size: .25 lbs. pork ribs

What's inside:

- BBQ sauce, sugar-free (.5 cup)
- Dry rib seasoning rub (1 package)
- Pepper
- Sat
- Pork ribs (1 lb.)

How to make:

1. Take out the slow cooker and heat it up.

2. While that heats up, use the seasoning, pepper, and salt to season up all the sides of the pork ribs.

3. Stand these ribs on the walls of your slow cooker, letting the bonier side of them face inside.

4. Pour the sauce on all sides, making sure that you have enough to coat.

5. Place the lid on the slow cooker and let this cook. After four hours, it's ready to serve.

Nutrients:

- Fat: 35g
- Protein: 34g
- Carbs: 2.5g
- Net carbs: 2.5g

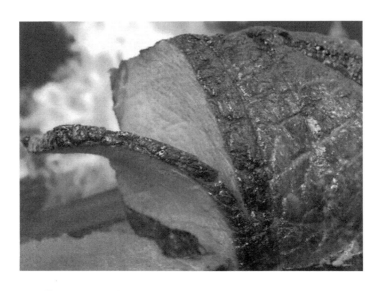

Kalua Pork Surprise

Servings: 4

Serving Size: .25 lbs. pork roast

What's inside:

- Chopped cabbage (.5 head)
- Water (.5 cup)
- Smoked paprika (1 Tbsp.)
- Pepper
- Salt
- Pork butt roast, boneless (1 lb.)

How to make:

1. You will need to bring out your slow cooker and get it all heated up for this recipe.

2. Season the pork with your smoked paprika, pepper, and salt before placing it into the slow cooker. Use the water to surround the pork.

3. Cover this up and cook it on a low setting. It is going to take about seven hours.

4. After this time, take the roast out of the slow cooker and put onto a plate. Add the cabbage to the bottom of the slow cooker and then add the pork roast back on top.

5. Cover the slow cooker again and let both these ingredients cook for another hour.

6. Take the pork roast out at this time and shred it up. Serve this with the cooked cabbage and some of the reserved liquid in the slow cooker before enjoying.

Nutrients:

- Fat: 20g
- Protein: 19g
- Carbs: 5g
- Net Carbs: 2.5g

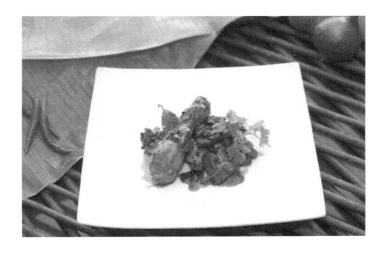

A Taste of French Pork Chops

Servings: 2

Serving Size: 1 pork chop

What's inside:

- Sour cream (.33 cup)
- Whipping cream, heavy (.33 cup)
- Blue cheese, crumbled up (.33 cup)
- Butter (2 Tbsp.)
- Pepper
- Salt
- Pork chops (2)

How to make:

1. Grab the pork chops and pat them nice and dry before seasoning with the salt and the pepper.

2. Now, heat up the butter until it is nice and warm in a skillet. When the butter is hot, add in the pork chops, making sure to sear them on each side for a bit.

3. Move the pork chops over to a plate and then let them rest a few minutes to cool down.

4. In a pan, you can melt the blue cheese. Make sure the heat isn't too high and that you keep on stirring to help prevent burning.

5. When the cheese has melted, add in some sour cream and the cream. Let these ingredients simmer together for a bit making sure to stir the whole time.

6. Add in some of the juice from the pork chops and let it continue to simmer while the pork chops rest.

7. Place the pork chops onto two plates and then pour your blue cheese over them before serving.

Nutrients:

- Fat: 34g
- Protein: 41 g
- Carbs: 4g
- Net Carbs: 4g

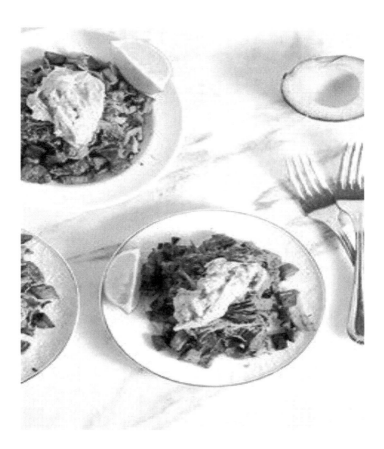

Carnitas

Servings: 4
Serving size: .25 lbs. pork roast

What's inside:

- Juice from a lime (1)
- Pepper
- Salt
- Diced onion (.5)
- Minced garlic clove (2)
- Pork butt roast, boneless (1 lb.)
- Olive oil (1 Tbsp.)
- Chili powder (.5 Tbsp.)

How to make:

1. Take out your slow cooker and let it preheat on a low setting.

2. While that warms up, mix together the olive oil and the chili powder. Use these ingredients to help season the pork and rub it all over.

3. Add the pork into the heated up slow cooker, making sure that the fat side is up.

4. Top the pork with the lime juice, pepper, salt, onion, and garlic.

5. Place the lid on top of the slow cooker and keep it on a low setting. It will need to cook for 8 hours.

6. Move the pork over to a cutting board. Shred up the meat using a fork and then serve warm.

Nutrients:

- Fat: 13g
- Protein: 23g
- Carbs: 3g
- Net Carbs: 2g

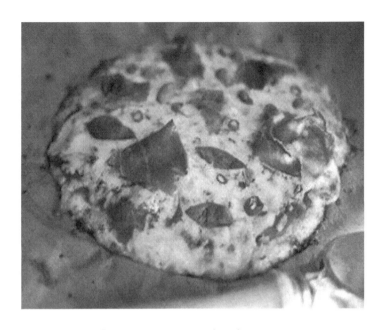

Low Carb Pepperoni Pizza

Servings: 2

Serving Size: 1 Tortilla

What's inside:

- Pepperoni (.5 cup)
- Dried Italian seasoning (2 tsp.)
- Mozzarella cheese (1 cup)
- Tomato sauce (4 Tbsp.)
- Tortillas, low carb (2)

- Olive oil (2 Tbsp.)

How to make:

1. Take out a skillet and heat up the olive oil. Add in the tortillas.

2. Spoon your chosen tomato sauce over the tortillas and properly spread it over the tortilla.

3. Sprinkle on the cheese, pepperoni, and Italian seasoning. Remember that you need to work quickly here to make sure that the tortillas don't burn while you do.

4. Cook these for a few minutes to make the tortilla crispy on the bottom.

5. When the tortillas are cooked, move over to your cutting board and slice up. Place onto a serving plate and enjoy.

Nutrients:

- Fat: 44g
- Protein: 27g

- Carbs: 17g
- Net Carbs: 8g

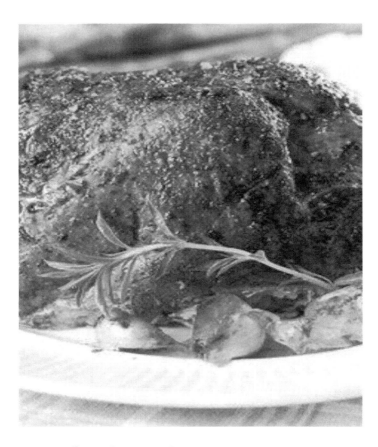

Grandma's Beef Roast

Servings: 4
Serving size: 25 beef roast

What's inside:

- Broccoli (1 bag)
- Toasted sesame oil (1 tsp.)
- Soy sauce (.25 cup)
- Beef broth (.5 cup)
- Pepper
- Salt
- Beef chuck roast (1 lb.)

How to make:

1. This recipe is going to need the slow cooker out. Make sure it has time to heat up to the low setting.

2. Take out your cutting board and place the chuck roast on it. Season the roast with your pepper and salt before thinly slicing the roast.

3. Add the slices of beef into the slow cooker. Take out a small bowl and mix together the sesame oil, soy sauce, and beef broth. Pour this mixture on top of the beef.

4. Cover the slow cooker and cook these ingredients on a low setting for 4 hours.

5. After this time is done, you can add in the frozen broccoli as well as a bit more beef broth if needed. Cook a bit longer and then serve this dish warm.

Nutrients:

- Fat: 24g
- Protein: 30g
- Carbs: 9g
- Net Carbs: 6g

Keto Friendly Potato Skins

Servings: 3

Serving Size: 1 bell pepper

What's inside:

- Ghee (1 Tbsp.)
- Sour cream (.25 cup)
- Avocado (1)
- Shredded cheese (.5 cup)
- Bell peppers, favorite color (3)
- Pepper
- Salt
- Ground beef (.5 lb.)

How to make:

1. Turn on the oven and let it heat up to 400 degrees. While that heats up, line a baking sheet with some foil.

2. In a skillet, melt the ghee. When it is hot enough, you can add in the ground beef, taking the time to season it with the pepper and the salt as well.

3. Stir the ground beef around, breaking up the chunks. Keep cooking until you see the beef is completely done.

4. While the beef is cooking, slice the bell peppers to make your potato skins. Cut off the top of each, slice it in half, and pull out all the ribs and the seeds. Cut until you get your desired bell pepper boat shape.

5. Place these peppers on your baking sheet. Spoon the beef into these peppers and sprinkle with some cheese on top. Place into the oven to bake for a bit.

6. After ten minutes, take them out of the oven. In the meantime, mix the sour cream and avocado together until smooth.

7. Divide up the peppers between three plates and top with the avocado cream before serving:

Nutrients:

- Fat: 30g
- Protein: 26g

- Carbs: 15g
- Net Carbs: 8g

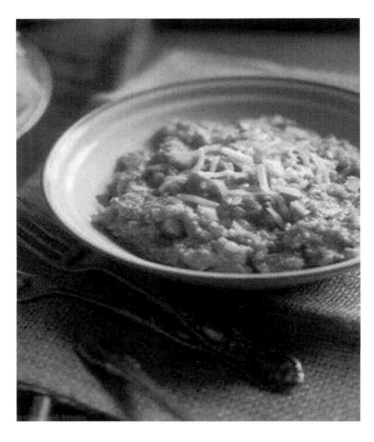

Double Cheeseburger Bacon Casserole

Servings: 8

Serving size: 1/8th of the casserole

What's inside:

- Ground beef and bacon part
- Pepper
- Salt
- Ground beef (1 lb.)
- Ghee (1 Tbsp.)
- Bacon (1 lb.)
- Casserole part
- Pepper
- Salt
- Shredded cheese (.75 cup)
- Beaten eggs (4)
- Whipping cream, heavy (.5 cup)
- Ghee (1 Tbsp.)

How to make:

1. We will start with the beef and bacon part in here. Take out a skillet and let the bacon cook on both sides to make it nice and crispy. Move this to a plate lined with paper towels and then cool it down for five minutes. Move to a cutting board and chop.

2. In a second separate skillet, heat up the ghee until it is nice and warm. Add in the ground beef and season with the pepper and salt.

3. Cook the meat until it is browned, making sure to break up any of the chunks of beef that are there. Drain out the fat from the meat and mix with the bacon.

4. Now, you can work on the casserole. Turn on the oven and let it heat up to 350 degrees. Use the ghee to grease up your baking dish.

5. Spoon this bacon and meat mixture into the baking dish to make the first layer.

6. Take out a bowl and mix together half the cheese, the eggs, and the cream. Season this with some pepper and salt before pouring on top of the meat. Top with the rest of the cheese.

7. Place the casserole dish into the oven. After 30 minutes, you can take it out.

8. Allow the casserole some time to cool down, about five minutes, before you slice it up and serve.

Nutrients:

- Fat: 45g
- Protein: 40g
- Carbs: 1.5g
- Net Carbs: 1.5g

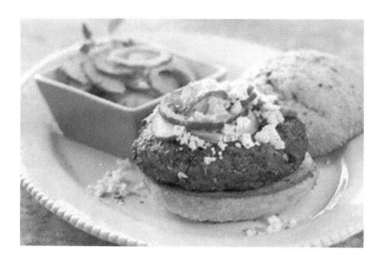

Zeus Burgers

Serves: 2

Serving Size: 6 oz. patty

What's inside:

- Ghee: (1 Tbsp.)
- Feta cheese (2 oz.)
- Ground beef (6 oz.)
- Ground lamb (6 oz.)
- Pepper
- Salt
- Dijon mustard (1 Tbsp.)

- Sliced scallion, both the green and white parts (1)
- Chopped mint leaves (2 Tbsp.)

How to make:

1. To start this recipe, bring out a bowl and combine the mustard, scallion, and mint leaves. Season with some pepper and salt.

2. Add in the ground beef and the ground lamb to this bowl and then form this into four patties.

3. Place the feta cheese and patties in between the burger buns. Pinch up the edges of the burgers to seal them in.

4. Now, you need to heat up a skillet with some of the ghee. When the skillets are hot, add on the burger patties and cook for about 5 minutes on both sides. Serve warm.

Nutrients:

- Fat: 48g
- Protein: 41g

- Carbs: 2g
- Net Carbs: 2g

Vegan and Vegetarian Meals

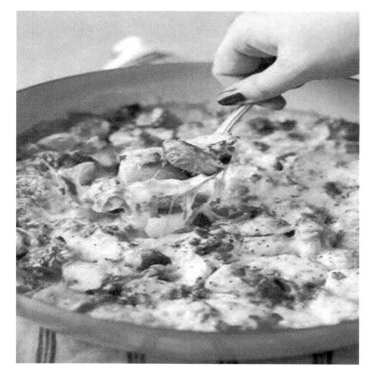

Cheesy Brussel Sprouts

Serves: 2

Serving Size: ½ soup

What's inside:

- Olive oil (2 Tbsp.)
- Cream cheese (.75 cup)
- Minced garlic cloves (4)
- Brussels Sprouts (25)
- Salt
- Pepper
- Lemon juice (2 tsp.)

How to make:

1. Take the Brussels sprouts and rinse them off in cold water before removing the stems.

2. Take out a skillet and heat up your olive oil on it. Add in the garlic and the sprouts to the pan and let them cook to make it tender.

3. Add in the lemon juice and cream cheese and cook until they are warmed up.

4. Move these to two bowls and then serve.

Nutrients:

- Fat: 18.5g
- Protein: 10g
- Carbs: 12g.
- Net carbs: 8g

A Taste of Italian Noodles

Servings: 3

Serving Size: .75 cup

What's inside:

- Mashed garlic cloves (4)
- Olive oil (4 Tbsp.)
- Zucchini noodles (2 cups)
- Chopped basil (3 Tbsp.)
- Pepper
- Salt
- Chopped red pepper, bell (.5)
- Red pepper flakes (1 tsp.)

How to make:

1. Start by bringing out the spiralizer and turning your zucchini into noodles. Set to the side.

2. Heat up your oil on a frying pan before adding in the red pepper, red pepper flakes, and garlic.

3. Cook these ingredients for a few minutes. Then, you can add in the zucchini noodles.

4. After another three minutes, move these to a plate and garnish with some basil before serving.

Nutrients:

- Fat: 15.6g
- Protein: 4g
- Carbs: 5.6g
- Net Carbs: 3g

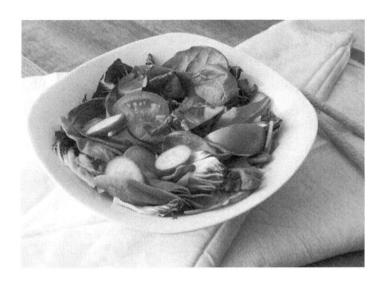

Summer Salad

Servings: 8

Serving Size: 1 cup.

What's inside:

- Olive oil (4 Tbsp.)
- Artichokes (8)
- Asparagus stalks (20)
- Salt
- Pepper
- Lemon juice (1)
- Green onions (4 tsp.)

- Egg white (1)
- Pistachio nuts (1 oz.)
- Chopped garlic cloves (2)

How to make:

1. Take out your pot and fill it about ¾ full of water. Add in a bit of lemon juice and salt.

2. Trim up the artichokes by getting rid of the leaves and then set the hearts to the side.

3. Place these leaves in the boiling water and let the cook. After 45 minutes, rinse these under cold water.

4. Place the artichokes into a food processor. Add in the egg white, garlic, green onions, pistachios, pepper, salt, half a glass of water, and lemon juice to this.

5. Blend the ingredients together for a few minutes. Slowly add and blend in the olive oil.

6. Cut up the artichokes and then arrange them on eight plates. Drizzle some of the sauce over the top of the artichokes.

7. Garnish with green onions before you serve.

Nutrients:

- Fat: 12g
- Protein: 21g
- Carbs: 5g
- Net Carbs: 3g

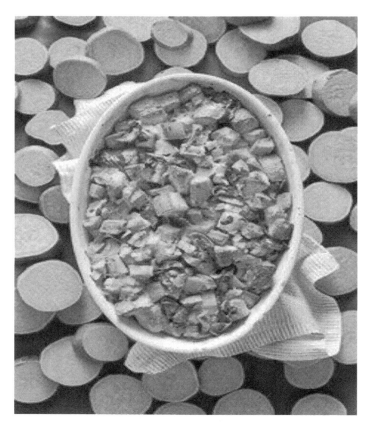

Sweet Potato Casserole

Servings: 4

What's inside:

- Spinach and kale mixture (4 cups)
- Coconut oil (.5 tsp.)

- Eggs (8)
- Seasonings of your choice
- Pepper
- Salt
- Nutmeg (.25 tsp.)
- Garlic powder (1 tsp.)
- Coconut milk (.25 cup)
- Chopped green onion (1)
- Diced sweet potatoes (2)

How to make:

1. Turn on the oven and let it heat up to 400 degrees. Grease up a casserole dish with some coconut oil.

2. In a big bowl, whisk together the eggs before adding in the greens, seasonings, coconut milk, sweet potato, and green onions.

3. Pour this mixture into your casserole dish and then add it to the oven to bake.

4. After 45 minutes, take the dish out of the oven. Cover up this dish with some foil and put it back into the oven.

5. After another 15 minutes, the casserole is done. You can take it from the oven and slice it up before serving.

Nutrients:

- Fat: 12g
- Protein: 14g
- Carbs: 11g
- Net carbs: 9g

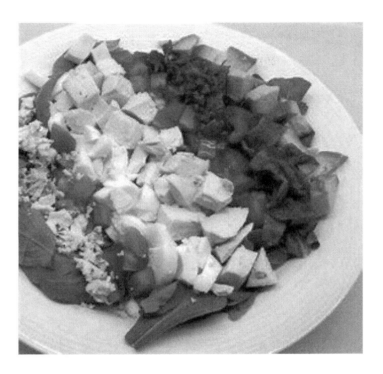

Living Easy Cobb Salad

Servings: 2

Serving Size: 1.5 cup

What's inside:

- Chopped hard-boiled eggs (2)
- Diced tomato (1)
- Chopped cucumber (1)
- Chopped spinach (2 cups)

135

- Chopped avocado (1)
- Cooked bacon slices (4)

How to make:

1. Bring out a serving platter and arrange the spinach on it in any way that you would like.

2. Top the spinach with the rest of the ingredients.

3. Serve and enjoy with your choice of ketogenic dressing.

Nutrients:

- Fat: 23g
- Protein: 31g
- Carbs: 6g
- Net Carbs: 6g

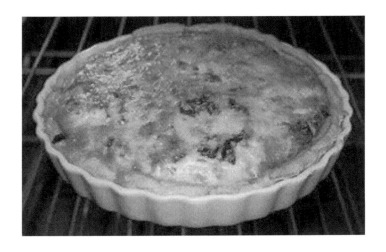

Feta Mushroom Quiche

Servings: 6

Serving Size: 1/6th Quiche

What's inside:

- Pepper
- Salt
- Mozzarella (.5 cup)
- Parmesan (.25 cup)
- Feta cheese (2 oz.)
- Milk (1 cup)
- Eggs (4)
- Spinach (10 oz.)

- Minced garlic cloves (1)
- Sliced button mushrooms (8 oz.)

How to make:

1. Turn on the oven and let it heat up to 400 degrees. Take your spinach and squeeze out any extra water.

2. Heat up about a tablespoon of the oil in a skillet and then add in the mushrooms and garlic. Cook until tender for about seven minutes.

3. Now, you will need to prepare a pie dish. Grease it up with some cooking spray and place the spinach along the bottom.

4. When the spinach is laid, pour the garlic and mushrooms over the spinach and top with the feta cheese.

5. In another bowl, whisk together the parmesan cheese, eggs, and milk. Season just a bit with some pepper before pouring this over the ingredients in your pie diet.

6. Make sure to sprinkle on some mozzarella all over it.

7. Place the pie dish onto a baking tray and then into the oven. After 45 minutes, this quiche should be done.

8. Take the dish out of the oven and allow it a few minutes to cool down before you serve.

Nutrients:

- Fat: 18g
- Protein: 17g
- Carbs: 4g
- Net Carbs: 1g

Dairy-Free Meals

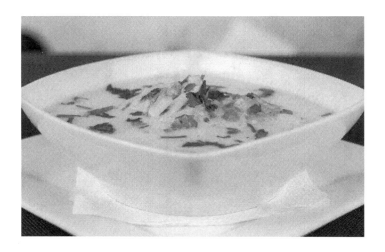

Cream of Chicken Soup

Servings: 4

Serving Size: 1 cup

What's inside:

- Onion powder (2 tsp.)
- Almond milk (1.33 cup)
- Chopped chicken thighs (.5 cup)
- Dried thyme (.25 tsp.)
- Pepper
- Salt (1 tsp.)

- Chicken broth (2 cups)
- Cauliflower (2)
- Collagen protein beef gelatin (.5 cup)
- Celery seeds (.25 tsp.)
- Garlic powder (.5 tsp.)

How to make:

1. Add all the ingredients except the gelatin and chicken into a big soup pot. Place it on medium heat and add the lid and let the ingredients boil.

2. Lower the heat once they start boiling and then continue to simmer until the cauliflower is soft.

3. Turn the heat off. Take out a cup of this liquid and boil it along with the gelatin. Whisk until the gelatin is dissolved. When finished, pour it into a big blender.

4. Add in the cooked cauliflower mixture and blend to make it smooth and creamy. Pour everything back into the pot and place it on low heat.

5. Add in the chicken and then stir. Cover and cook until it is all warm and then serve when ready.

Nutrients:

- Fat: 21g
- Protein: 22g
- Carbs: 5g
- Net Carbs: 2g

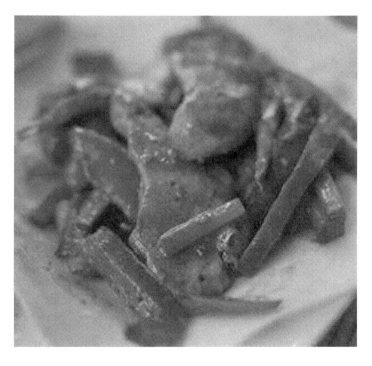

Thai Chicken Skillet

Servings: 6

Serving Size: .75 cup (1 chicken thigh)

What's inside:

- Cauliflower rice to serve
- Thai curry paste (2 Tbsp.)
- Pepper
- Coconut milk (1.5 cups)

- Lime juice (3 Tbsp.)
- Chopped green bell pepper (9 oz.)
- Minced garlic cloves (3)
- Chopped onion (.5 cup)
- Chicken thighs (6)
- Chicken stock (1.5 cups)
- Coconut oil (3 Tbsp.)

Toppings:

- Chopping cilantro (1 handful)
- Sliced red chili pepper
- Lime juice

How to make:

1. Take out a skillet and turn it on high heat. Add in a bit of oil and let it heat up. Add in the chicken when the oil is ready, making sure it stays in one layer.

2. Lower the heat a bit and then cook the chicken for the next five minutes. After that time is done, flip the chicken over and let it cook for another three minutes.

3. Now, you can use a slotted spoon and take the chicken out of the skillet. Place the chicken on a plate.

4. Add the rest of the oil to the skillet and then cook the garlic and the onion. After a few minutes, add the bell pepper and the rest of the ingredients into the skillet.

5. A few minutes later, put the chicken back into the skillet. These all need to cook for another 10 minutes.

6. Move this skillet to a preheated oven. Broil for a few minutes to make it crispy. Top with the optional toppings and then serve with some cauliflower rice on the side.

Nutrients:

- Fat: 11g
- Protein: 18g
- Carbs; 12g
- Net Carbs: 8g

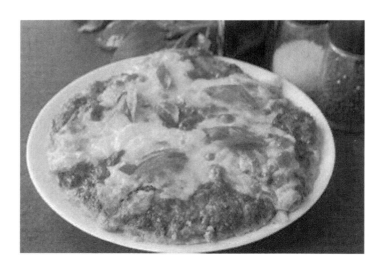

Italian Meatza

Servings: 8

Serving Size: 1/8th Meatza

What's inside:

- Basil, chopped
- Minced garlic cloves (2)
- Pepper (1 tsp.)
- Salt (1 tsp.)
- Dried Italian herbs (5 Tbsp.)
- Basil (2 Tbsp.)
- Ground beef (2 lbs.)

Topping

- Artichoke heart (1)
- Sliced olives (10)
- Sliced red bell pepper (1)
- Sliced sun-dried tomatoes (.5 cup)
- Tomato sauce (1 cup)
- Arugula leaves (1 cup)

How to make:

1. Start by making the crust. Bring out a bowl and mix together all the ingredients that are needed for the crust.

2. Add this mixture either onto one large pie pan or two smaller ones and then press it into the bottom of the pan.

3. Turn on the oven and give it some time to heat up to 400 degrees. Place the pan inside and let it cook.

4. After 15 minutes, take the pan out of the oven and drain off the fat from the pan.

5. To make the toppings, spread out the tomato sauce over the crust and then sprinkle the rest over it.

6. Place this back into the oven for 10 minutes until done. You can slice it into wedges before serving.

Nutrients:

- Fat: 31g
- Protein: 25g
- Carbs: 3g
- Net carbs: 1g

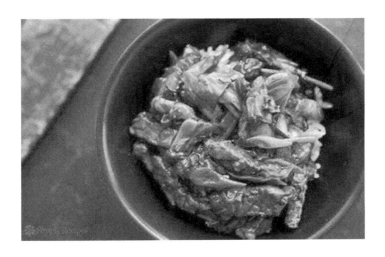

Steak and Broccoli Stir Fry

Servings: 4

Serving size: 1 cup

What's inside:

- Pumpkin seeds (2 Tbsp.)
- Sliced yellow onion (2)
- Sliced rib eye steaks (1.5 lbs.)
- Pepper
- Salt
- Tamari sauce (2 Tbsp.)
- Chopped broccoli (18 oz.)
- Coconut oil (8 oz.)

How to make:

1. Bring out a wok and place it over medium heat. Add in half of your oil and heat it up.

2. When the oil is heated, add in the slices of steak and cook, so they become browned. Sprinkle on the pepper and salt and mix them around well.

3. Use a slotted spoon to take the steaks from the wok and place onto a plate to cool down.

4. Add in the onions and broccoli and cook to until the vegetables are tender. Add in some more oil if needed.

5. Now, add in the tamari before throwing the steak back into the pan as well. Adjust the seasonings if needed.

6. Serve this warm with some pumpkin seeds.

Nutrients:

- Fat: 34g
- Protein: 19g

- Carbs: 7g
- Net Carbs: 6g

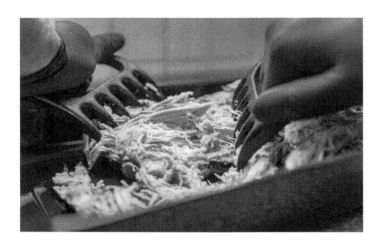

Spicy Pulled Pork

Servings: 3

Serving Size: .33 lbs. pork

What's inside:

- Olive oil (1 Tbsp.)
- Salt (.5 Tbsp.)
- Cayenne pepper (.25 tsp.)
- Pepper powder (.25 Tbsp.)
- Anise seeds (.25 tsp.)
- Ground ginger (.25 tsp.)
- Cocoa nibs (.5 Tbsp.)
- Pork shoulder (1 lb.)

How to make:

1. Process all the cocoa nibs and spices together in a grinder.

2. Rub this new mixture all over your pork. Add the pork to a baking dish.

3. Turn on the oven and let it heat up to 400 degrees. When the oven is warm, add in the pork.

4. After a few hours, you can take it out. When the pork is done, set it on a cutting board and then shred using some forks.

5. Serve with a tomato salad. You can also leave the pork in a slow cooker on low setting for eight hours if you prefer.

Nutrients:

- Fat: 24g
- Protein: 22g
- Carbs: 6g
- Net Carbs: 6g

Ground Pork Tacos

Servings: 6

Serving Size: 5 wraps

What's inside:

- Pepper (.5 tsp.)
- Salt (1 tsp.)
- Garlic powder (1.5 tsp.)
- Lettuce leaves (20)
- Cumin (1 tsp.)
- Onion powder (1.5 tsp.)
- Ground pork (2 lbs.)

Toppings

- Red bell pepper, chopped (.75 cup)
- Chopped green bell pepper (.75 cup)
- Chopped onions (2)
- Salsa (.25 cup)

How to make:

1. Add the onion powder, pepper, salt, cumin, garlic powder, and pork to a bowl. Use your hands to mix them well.

2. Place the skillet on medium heat before adding in the meat mixture. Make sure to stir the whole time that it is cooking until it turns brown.

3. Use a spoon to remove the pork and leave it in a bowl. Let the remaining fat stay in the skillet.

4. Add the salsa and mix well. Taste and see if you need more seasonings in it.

5. Lay the lettuce leaves on the working area. Place a bit of the pork filling in the center.

6. Sprinkle the onions and both peppers on top and then wrap up the tacos before serving.

Nutrients:

- Fat: 21g
- Protein: 16g
- Carbs: 11g
- Net Carbs: 10g

Chapter 8:
"Super-Fast Keto" – Quick and Easy Emergency Keto Meal Ideas

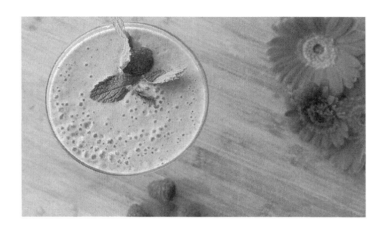

Berry Smoothie

Servings: 2

Serving Size: 10 oz.

What's inside:

- Liquid stevia (.25 tsp.)
- Ice cubes (.5 cup)
- Berries (.5 cup)
- Spinach (1 cup)
- Avocado (.5)

- Peaches and cream ketone powder (1 scoop)
- Coconut milk (1 cup)

How to make:

1. Take out a blender and combine together all of the ingredients.

2. Blend all these together thoroughly until it becomes frothy and well combined.

3. Pour into two glasses and enjoy.

Nutrients:

- Fat: 40g
- Protein: 4g.
- Carbs: 16g
- Net Carbs: 8g

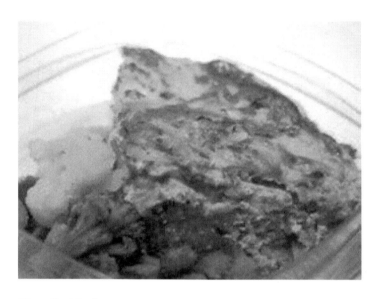

Pork Frittata

Servings: 4

Serving size: ¼ frittata

What's inside:

- Sliced prosciutto (2 oz.)
- Chopped pancetta (4 oz.)
- Pepper
- Salt
- Whipping cream (1 cup)
- Eggs (8)

- Butter (1 Tbsp.)
- Dill, chopped (1 Tbsp.)

How to make:

1. Allow the oven time to heat up to 375 degrees. Prepare a baking pan and grease it with butter.

2. Bring out a bowl and whisk the cream and eggs together. Season with some pepper and salt and whisk.

3. Pour this egg mixture into your pan and then sprinkle the pancetta to distribute throughout.

4. Tear the pieces of prosciutto and place on top before sprinkling on the dill. Put into the oven.

5. The edges should be golden after 25 minutes. You can now it take out of the pan. Slice up into four servings and serve.

Nutrients:

- Fat: 39g
- Protein: 21g

- Carbs: 3g
- Net Carbs: 3g

Sausage Stacks

Servings: 2

Serving Size: 1 Stack

What's inside:

- Pepper
- Salt
- Avocado (1)
- Eggs (2)
- Ghee (2 Tbsp.)
- Onion powder (.5 tsp.)
- Garlic powder (.5 tsp.)
- Ground pork (8 oz.)

How to make:

1. Turn on the oven and let it heat up to 375 degrees. While that warms up, throw the onion powder, garlic powder, and ground pork in a bowl. Form this into two patties.

2. Heat up a tablespoon of ghee in the skillet and add the patties. Cook these until browned.

3. Move the patties to the baking sheet and cook in the oven. After ten minutes, take these out and let them cool down.

4. Add the rest of your ghee to the skillet. Once it heats up, add the eggs into the skillet and cook for three minutes.

5. While those cook, you can mash up the avocado. Season the eggs with the pepper and salt.

6. Take the patties from the oven and place onto two plates. Spread half the avocado on top of each patty. Top with the egg and then serve hot.

Nutrients:

- Fat: 44g
- Protein: 29g
- Carbs: 7g
- Net Carbs 3g

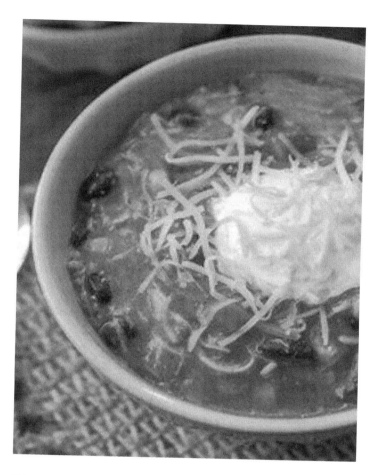

Taco Soup

Serves: 4

Serving Size: 2 cups

What's inside:

- Chicken broth (3.5 cups)
- Ground beef (2 lbs.)
- Tomato puree (.5 cup)
- Cheddar cheese (1 cup)
- Cream cheese (1 cup)

How to make:

1. Take out your slow cooker and get it all set up.

2. Add in the chicken broth, ground beef, tomato puree, cheese, cream cheese, and some salt to taste.

3. Cover the slow cooker and turn it to a low setting.

4. Cook for four hours on the low setting before serving.

Nutrients:

- Fat: 20g
- Protein: 21g

- Carbs: 6g
- Net Carbs: 4.8g

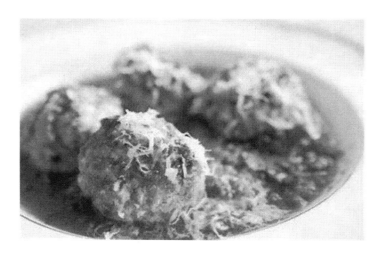

Tomato Meatballs:

Serves: 4

Serving Size: 2 cups

What's inside:

- Canned tomatoes (2 cups)
- Diced garlic (2 cloves)
- Diced onion (1)
- Olive oil (2 Tbsp.)
- Salt
- Dried oregano (1 tsp.)
- Onion powder (1 tsp.)
- Garlic powder (1 tsp.)

166

- Ground beef (1.3 lbs.)

How to make:

1. Take out a bowl and mix together the salt, oregano, onion powder, garlic powder, and ground beef.

2. Form about 10 meatballs from this mixture.

3. Now you will need your Instant Pot. Choose the sauté function and then add in the garlic, onion, and olive oil. These need to cook for the next five minutes.

4. Afterward, add in the meatballs and the tomato sauce and mix them well together.

5. Lock the lid onto the pot and press Manual. Cook this on high pressure for a bit.

6. After five minutes, let the pressure release naturally and then serve.

Nutrients:

- Fat: 26.5g
- Protein: 46g
- Carbs: 8g
- Net Carbs: 4g

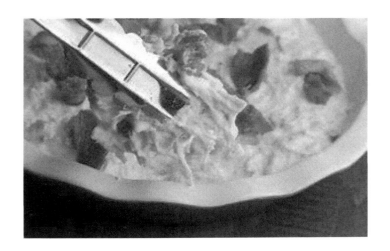

Crack Chicken

Serves: 4

Serving Size: 1 chicken breast

What's inside:

- Bacon slices, cooked (8)
- Cream cheese (16 oz.)
- Ranch dressing (1 packet)
- Chicken breast (4)

How to make:

1. Bring out your slow cooker and place the chicken inside.

2. Pour in the packet of ranch dressing and then add in the cream cheese as well.

3. Cover the slow cooker and let this cook on a low setting for eight hours or until chicken is done.

4. Right before the meal is done, cook up the bacon slices until crisp. Crumble them up and mix in with the chicken before you serve.

Nutrients:

- Fat: 23g
- Protein: 40g
- Carbs: 6g
- Net Carbs: 5g

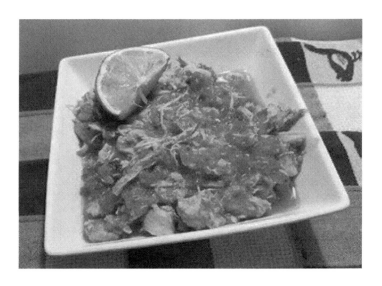

Salsa Chicken

Servings: 4

Serving Size: 1 chicken breast

What's inside:

- Shredded cheese (2 cups)
- Salsa (2 cups)
- Chicken breast (4)

How to make:

1. To start this recipe, bring out the slow cooker and grease it with some olive oil.

2. Place the chicken into the slow cooker and then pour the salsa on top.

3. Cover the slow cooker and cook this on a high setting. It will take two hours to cook.

4. When this is done, place the chicken into a baking dish and top with the cheese.

5. Turn the oven on to 425 degrees and put the baking dish inside. It will be done in 15 minutes. Serve and enjoy.

Nutrients:

- Fat: 18.3g
- Protein: 43g
- Carbs: 8g
- Net carbs: 4.2g

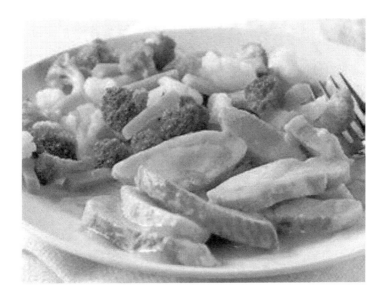

Turkey and Veggies

Servings: 6

Serving Size: 1.5 cups

What's inside:

- Canned tomatoes (14 oz.)
- Tomato sauce (1 cup)
- Vegetable broth (1 cup)
- Chopped zucchini (1 cup)
- Chopped bell pepper (1.5 cups)
- Minced garlic (2 tsp.)

- Chopped onion (1)
- Chili paste (1.5 Tbsp.)
- Ground turkey (1 lb.)
- Butter (1 Tbsp.)
- Olive oil (1 Tbsp.)

How to make:

1. Pour the olive oil and heat it up in the Instant Pot.

2. Cook the ground turkey until browned. Add the rest of the ingredients and mix well. Place the lid on the Instant Pot and then set it to a Manual setting.

3. Cook in high pressure for eight minutes and then quick-release. Serve.

Nutrients:

- Fat: 12g
- Protein: 20g
- Carbs: 2g
- Net Carbs: 1g

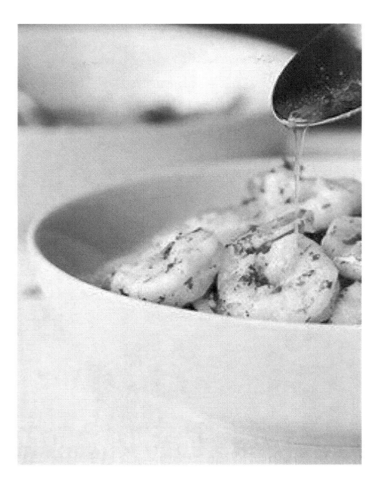

Shrimp Scampi

Servings: 2

Serving Size: .25 lbs. shrimp

What's inside:

- White cooking wine (.25 cup)
- Lemon juice (.5 Tbsp.)
- Butter (1 Tbsp.)
- Chicken broth .25 cup)
- Shrimp, raw (.5 lb.)

How to make:

1. You can bring out the slow cooker in order to get started on this recipe.

2. Add the shrimp, chicken broth, butter, lemon juice, and white cooking wine inside.

3. Add in some salt and pepper if you would like before placing the lid on top.

4. This needs to cook at a low setting for the next two and a half hours. Serve when done.

Nutrients:

- Fat: 15g
- Protein: 23g

- Carbs: 5g
- Net Carbs: 2g

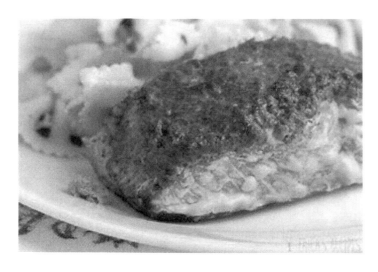

Salmon and Spinach Pesto

Servings: 4

Serving Size: 3 oz. Salmon

What's inside:

- Lemon juice (1 tsp.)
- Grated lemon zest (1 tsp.)
- Heavy cream (1.5 cups)
- Sliced smoked salmon (12 oz.)
- Low carb pasta (16 oz.)
- Butter (1 Tbsp.)
- Pepper

- Salt
- Olive oil (.5 cup)
- Grated Parmesan cheese (1 cup)
- Baby spinach (10 cups)
- Walnuts (.25 cup)
- Garlic cloves (2)

How to make:

1. To start, add in the pepper, salt, olive oil, parmesan, spinach, walnuts, and garlic into a food processor. Pulse these ingredients together until they are pureed.

2. Bring out the Instant Pot and turn it on to a manual setting. Pour in four cups of water and then add in the pasta and the butter.

3. Cover the pot and turn it onto the manual setting. This needs to cook on high pressure for the next four minutes.

4. When this time is done, release the pressure quickly. Keep the pot on a sauté setting.

5. Add in the remainder of your ingredients and then mix well. Let this mixture simmer for a few minutes before serving.

Nutrients:

- Fat: 60g
- Protein: 25g
- Carbs: 9g
- Net Carbs: 6g

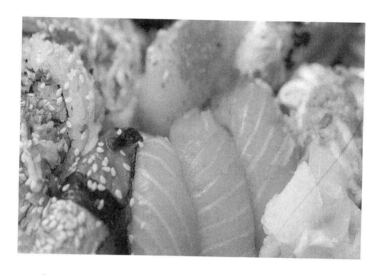

Asian Tuna

Serves: 2

Serving Size: 1 tuna fillet

What's inside:

- Pepper
- Salt
- Tuna fillets (2)
- Grated ginger (.25 tsp.)
- Coconut aminos (3 Tbsp.)
- Paprika (1 tsp.)
- Maple syrup (2 Tbsp.)

- Brown sugar (1 Tbsp.)
- Coconut oil (1 Tbsp.)

How to make:

1. Prepare and turn on your Instant Pot.

2. Add in the brown sugar and coconut oil. Cook until the sugar has dissolved.

3. Pour in the ginger, coconut aminos, paprika, and maple syrup. Mix well.

4. Add in the tuna fillets and then season with the pepper and salt. Cover the pot and set it on manual.

Chapter 9:
Common Mistakes Made By Meal Prepping Beginners and Intermediates

Before you get started with meal prepping, it is important to know that there are mistakes that can be made. This process is designed to be simple, but if you don't plan things out ahead of time and don't balance out your meals, it can get really difficult. Here are some of the most common mistakes that both beginners and intermediates to meal prepping make and how you can avoid them with your own journey.

- **Not hitting the grocery store to grab everything.**

This seems like something simple to remember, but it can make a big difference when it is time to prepare your meals. Trying to cook up your meals when you don't have all the ingredients that are needed can be frustrating. You will maybe try to find some substitutes, but often, you give up because you don't have the ingredients on hand.

To help avoid this, you should choose recipes that you want to use ahead of time. Then, write down all of the ingredients that you need before heading to the store. This can cut down on the stress when you are at the store, and ensures that you have every ingredient that you need when it is time to start cooking.

- **You don't include enough vegetables**

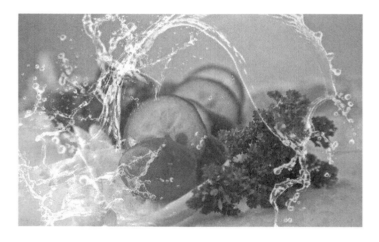

Meal prepping is a fantastic way for you to stick with a diet that is healthy, but it is also going to depend quite a lot on what you decide to prep ahead of time. A big mistake that you can make with meal planning is not adding in enough vegetables. You want to make sure that you stick with the right ratio of carbs for the ketogenic diet, but there are a ton of non-starchy vegetables that you can add into your meals.

These vegetables are so important. All the great nutrients inside them will help to keep you energized and can make losing weight easier. And these vegetables are great for filling you up, so you won't get as hungry in between meals. You should aim for a variety of vegetables and try to add in as many different colors to the meal as possible.

- **You don't balance the meals**

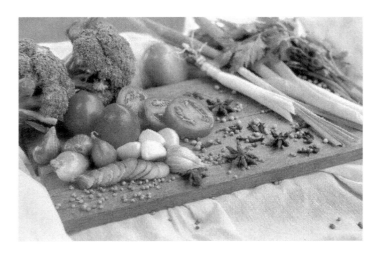

As you are working through the ketogenic diet, you need to make sure that you balance out your meals. If you just randomly throw some things together and call it a meal, how are you supposed to know if you are taking in enough of one nutrient or not enough of another one? Balancing your meals is so important when you are on the ketogenic diet and can make all the difference on whether you will actually see weight loss or not.

- **You make too much or too little**

When you are trying to meal prep for a few days, or even a few weeks ahead of time, it is sometimes hard to ensure you have the right number of servings. As someone who is new to the process, it is pretty common to either prep too much food at a time or too little. If you find that you are throwing out a lot of food at the end of the week, or you can't make the vegetables stretch long enough, then it is time to get a little more organized with your work.

Before you get started with this, think about how many meals you are planning to make and then determine the serving size of each before you start cooking. This can help to cut down on some prep time because all your stuff is sorted out. Make sure that you have enough servings of everything, but not too much, so that you get all the nutrients your body needs without all the waste.

- **Eating the same meals all the time**

You will find that it is really hard to stick with a meal plan if you keep eating the exact same meals every week. Sure, that can make things easier because you know exactly what you need to get, exactly how to cook it all, and exactly how much it will cost you. But most people do not want to eat the exact same thing all the time. This can get boring and isn't that much fun. If you are bored with your meal plan, it is much easier to give up. Some people like the consistency and don't mind eating the same meals all the time, but for most people, they like some variety.

The good news is that mixing up what you make doesn't have to be all that difficult. Some of the things that you can try include:

- Swap out the protein that you are using. Many dishes would taste unique if you switched chicken over to turkey

- Change up the spices and herbs you use.

- Add in some different vegetables.

You are not required to stick with the same meal for dinner and lunch just because you are on a meal plan. Take some time to experiment to see if there are any new combinations that you like that can keep your meal prepping healthy, exciting, and fresh.

- **You forget about the snacks**

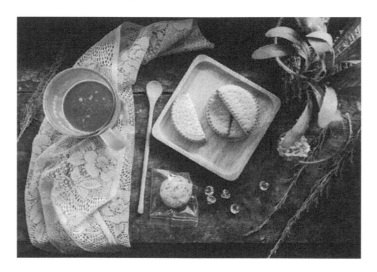

Many people who are just starting out with meal prepping will concentrate their efforts on breakfast, lunch, and dinner. But then, they forget about snacks. Most people eat snacks throughout the day, so not prepping these means that you may be tempted to reach for something unhealthy when you get hungry between meals. It is much better to include one or two snacks per day in your meal prepping to help you get the best results.

Getting started with meal prepping does not have to be difficult. Follow some of these tips to help you avoid the most common mistakes that beginners and intermediates make, and it won't be long before you become a professional meal prepper.

Chapter 10:
Bonus "Tips About Meal Prepping Your Way to Success

This guidebook has taken some time to talk about meal prepping and all the good ways that it can benefit you. We have talked about how to get started, how to make some delicious meals, and even how to be successful with meal prepping no matter what level you are when you get started.

Remember that anyone is able to get started with meal prepping. As long as you have some recipes to work with and you make the meals ahead of time, you are going to be successful. And when you implement meal prepping along with the ketogenic diet, you are going to also see some great weight loss benefits at the same time.

In this bonus chapter, we are going to spend some time looking at a few more tips and tricks that you can follow in order to be really successful with meal prepping. These are simple tips and tricks that you can use at any time to ensure that you are on the right track to seeing some great success with meal prepping. Some of the best tips that you can follow when you are ready to start meal prepping will include:

- **Keep your recipes someplace safe**

As you spend more time working with meal prepping, you will find that there are a ton of recipes that you will accumulate. You may decide to throw out some of these recipes because you find they aren't that good, or you may keep a bunch of them. But what are you going to do with the ones that you decide to keep so that you can reuse them at a later time?

It is important to find a safe place to put these recipes. Otherwise, it may be impossible to find them again if you want to reuse them. You can keep them in a folder on your computer. You can choose to start your own recipe book and keep them in there. You can even find a folder or a notebook to hold the recipes in. You can pick the method that works the best for you, as long as the recipes are kept in a safe location to find later.

- **Ask for input from others**

You are not the only person who is going to be eating these recipes. Other family members will enjoy the breakfasts, lunches, dinners, and snacks as well. Why not ask their opinion on some of the meals that you make. Including the whole family together can make a difference. They will all feel more involved so they are more likely to eat the meals, and they may be able to come up with some good ideas to try out when you are a little bit stuck.

You can ask each person in your home if they have some favorite meals that they want to make sure that you cook at least on occasion. Ask them if they have heard about any snacks or other options that you can make to include on the list as well. You don't have to use this all of the time, but it is great to have some of those notes down so you can get ideas when you are stuck. You can also ensure that everyone in the family is getting things that they enjoy too.

- **Check out the weather**

The weather can sometimes influence what you are going to make each week. If you notice that there is going to be an unseasonably warm day after a long winter, maybe consider having a night of grilling out. If you notice that there is going to be a cool spell for a few days and fall is about to come, you can consider putting on some soups. Watching the weather can make it easier to figure out what you will be in the mood for and can even help you to come up with the meals that you want to eat.

For many people, the weather is going to dictate the things they are hungry for. If you are having a cooler day and you want soup, you may find that all the meals in your fridge are not going to satisfy you unless some of them are soup. Looking at the weather can really make a difference especially if you know what your body tends to react to.

- **Keep a meal journal**

A meal journal is a great way to keep all your thoughts and recipes organized. If you tried out something new and really liked it, you can go ahead and write it down in the journal along with some notes. If you changed up something in a recipe to make it better, you could write this down as well. Or if the whole family agreed that one recipe was not all that good, you need to write this information down as well.

The point of your meal journal is to help you out. You can write down whatever you would like to inside. No one but you will be able to see it. But this is where you can keep your notes about what is working, what isn't working, and what you would like to change.

- **Theme nights can make a difference**

Another idea that you can use is to have a theme night. Monday could be soups and salads, Tuesdays can be Taco night, Wednesday can be pasta, and so on. You can choose the themes that work for you.

This theme night can help make meal prepping a little bit easier on you. You already know what kind of meal you are going to make on each day. So now, you just have to find the recipe that you want to work with. It can keep you organized and just makes things easier when you are planning them out.

- **Be careful about overstocking the fridge**

When your fridge is too overstocked, it is easy to get overwhelmed by all the choices that you have. And when the fridge has too much in it, it becomes easy for things to get lost in the back and forgotten about. If you want meal prepping to work for you, you need to make sure that things don't have a chance to go bad.

You can keep the fridge light and airy and only keep a sensible and realistic amount of food inside. You can also keep a list of everything that is inside the fridge somewhere nearby so that you can remember what is there and what needs to be eaten.

- **Have a master list of recipes**

Sit down and think about some of the meals and recipes that you and your family enjoy. These should be recipes that are easy to prepare and won't require a ton of ingredients. Write these all down and keep them handy in a notebook or somewhere else.

You don't have to use these recipes all the time, but if you need some inspiration on occasion for your meal plan, then this would be the place where you can turn to. Remember that variety is really important when it comes to meal prepping, so you don't want to just eat those ten to twenty recipes all the time. However, they can be really helpful when you are working on your meal plan to throw a few in on occasion.

- **Check out your calendar when meal planning**

Before you get too far in your meal planning process, you should bring out your activity calendar and see what is on the agenda for that week. Do you have to work late sometime this week? Do you plan to go visit your in-laws over the weekend for dinner? Is there a soccer game or some other meeting for the kids that you need to go to?

You need to take all of these issues into consideration when planning your meals. Once you have an idea of the schedule you will be on for the rest of the week, it becomes much easier to plan. For example, if you are going to be late at the office one night, then you may want to make that a leftover night to keep things simple.

This can work no matter what you have going on in your family schedule for that whole week. If you are going to the in-laws for supper, then you can take the night off and not plan anything for supper that night. If you have a soccer game one night, prepare a slow cooker meal. There are so many options. Often, the schedule you have for the week can make it easier to plan out your meals and stay on track.

Meal prepping is one of the best things that you can do for your life. It helps to reduce the stress, keeps you on a diet plan, and helps you save money. Follow some of the tips above, as well as the tips in this guidebook, to get the results that you're looking for.

Conclusion

Thank you for making it through to the end of *Meal Prepping*. Let's hope it was informative and able to provide you with all of the tools you need to achieve your goals whatever they may be.

The next step is to get started with meal prepping for your own needs. Meal prepping is something that everyone is able to benefit from, and it is so easy to do. You just need to pick out the recipes that you want to go with (and check that they belong to a diet plan if you are following it), and then prepare the meals ahead of time. There are so many different options that you can go with, and with the time and money that it saves, meal prepping is soon going to become your favorite activity.

When you are ready to start using meal prepping to help you stick with the ketogenic diet and to help you lose weight in no time, make sure to take a look at this guidebook to help you get going.

Finally, if you found this book useful in any way, a review on Amazon is always appreciated! Thank you!

66648768R00113

Made in the USA
Columbia, SC
18 July 2019